Multidisciplinary Approach for Colorectal Cancer

Edited by Keun-Yeong Jeong

Published in London, United Kingdom

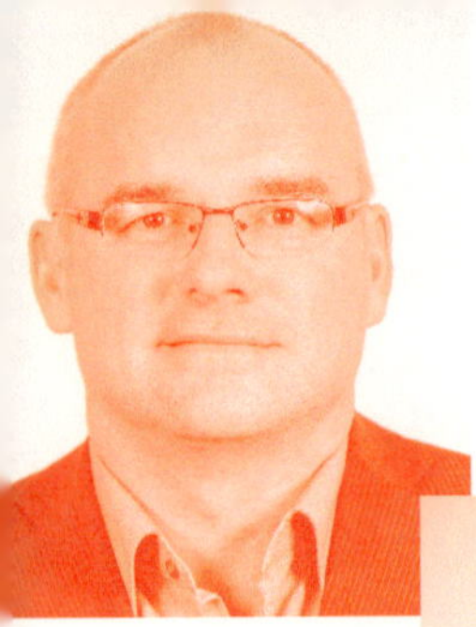
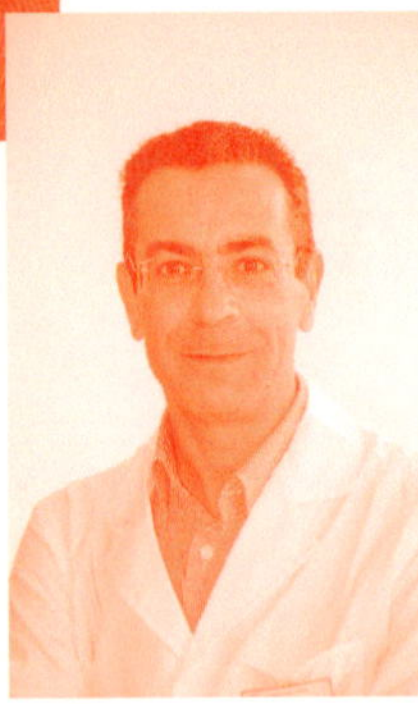
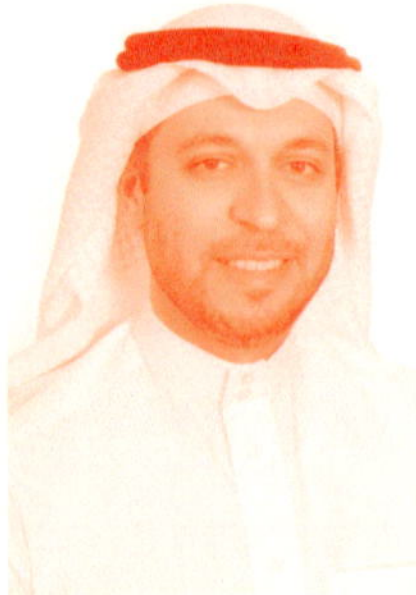
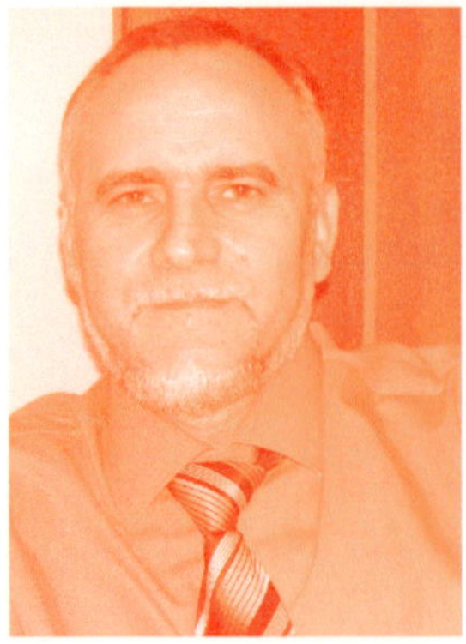
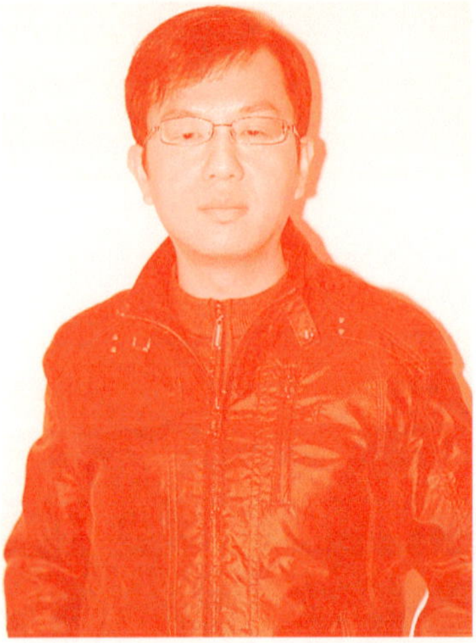
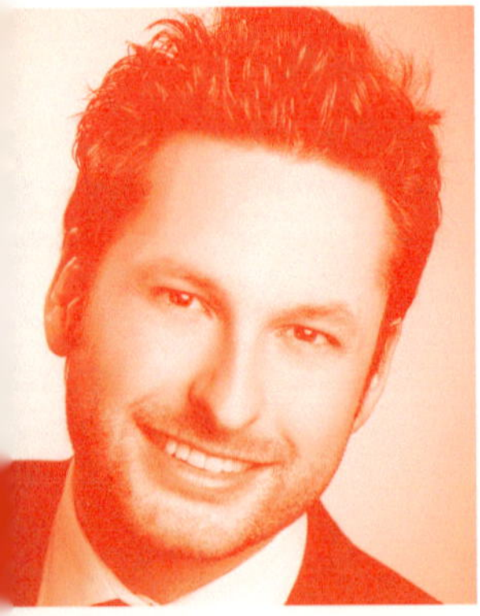
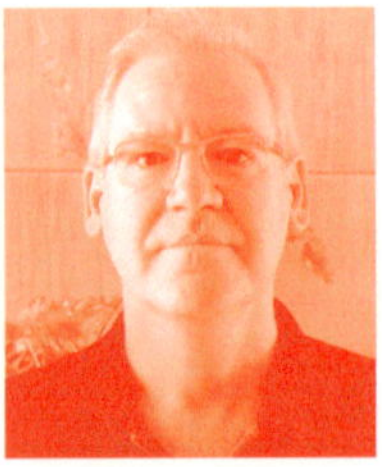

IntechOpen

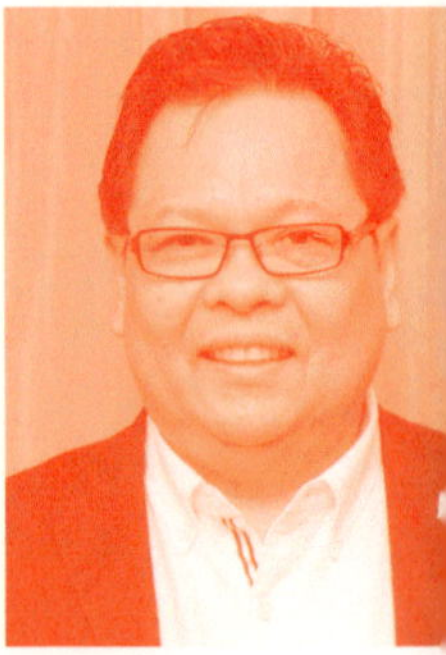
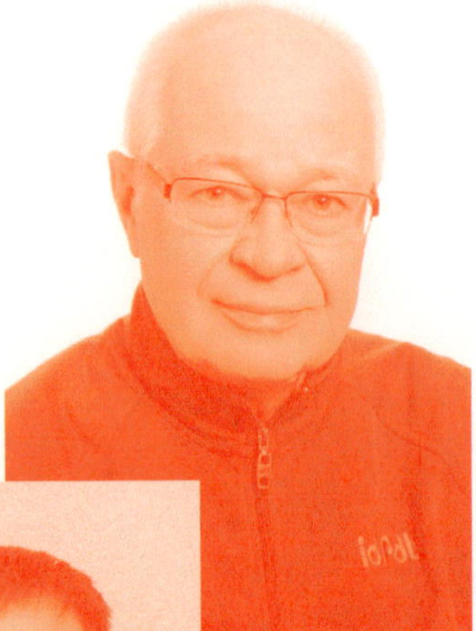
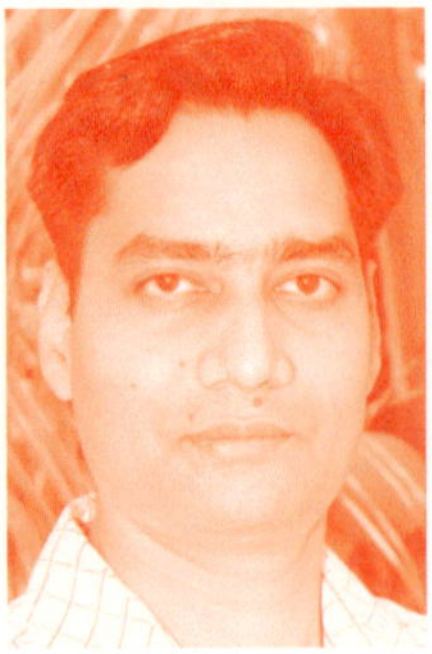
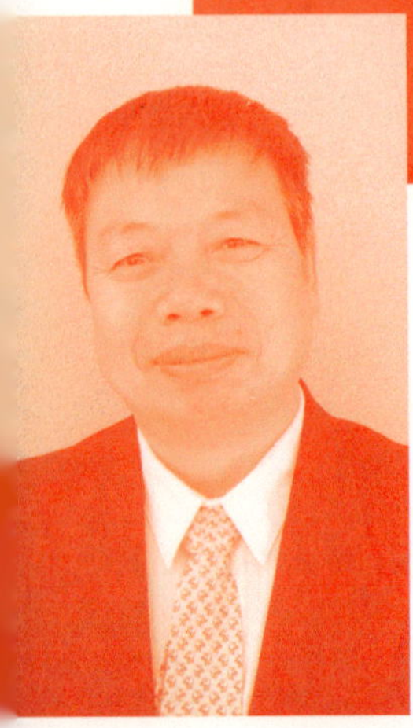
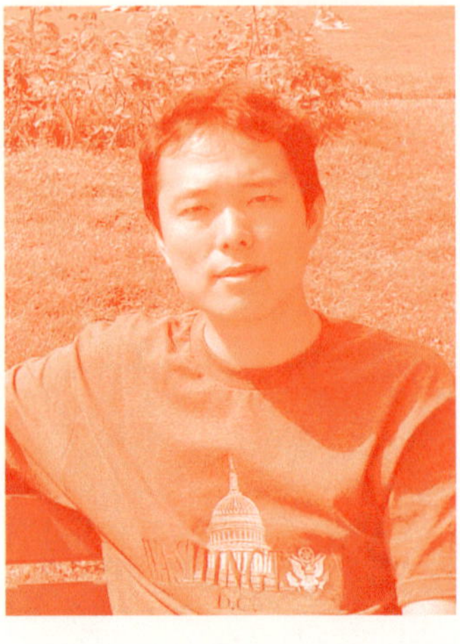
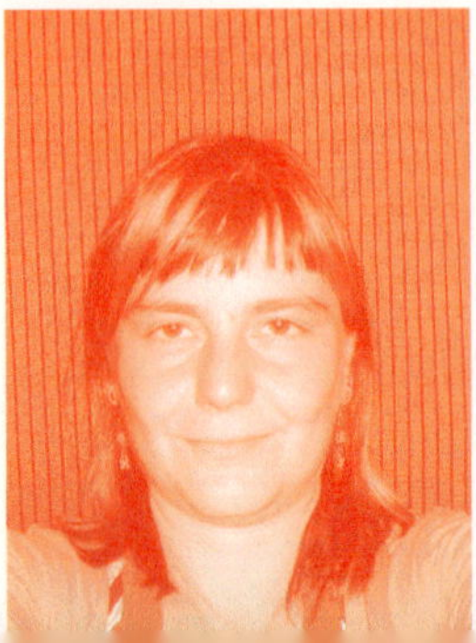

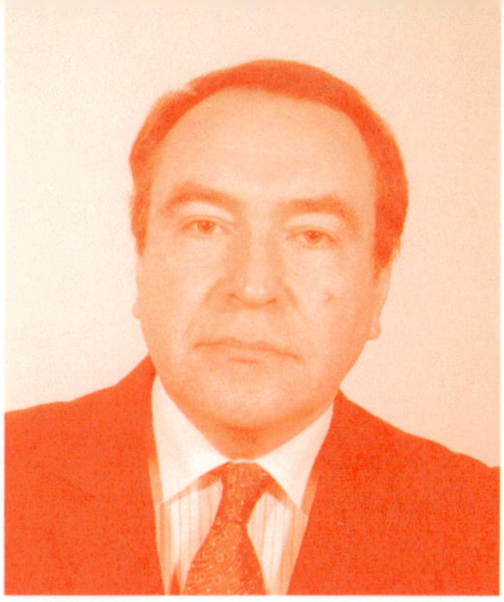
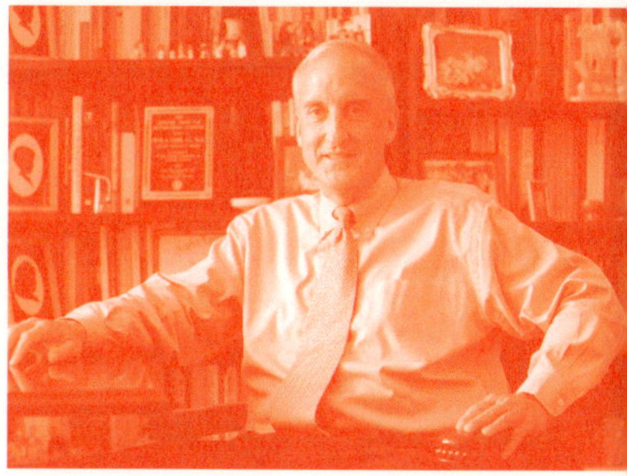
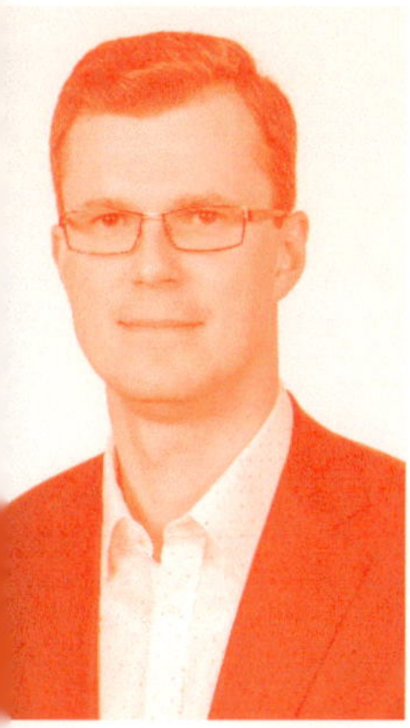
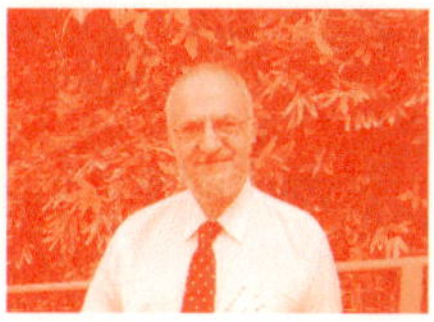
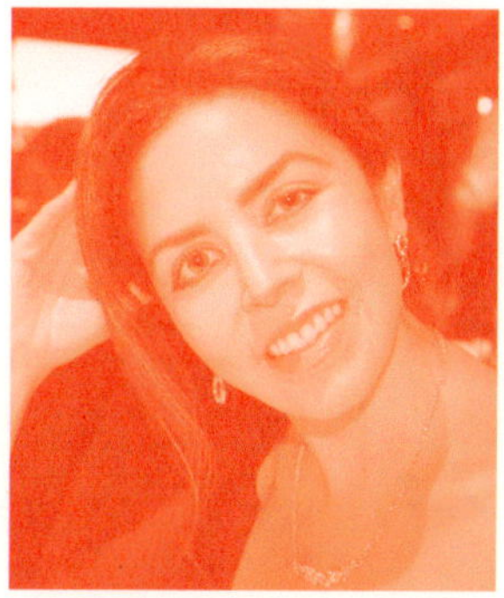

Supporting open minds since 2005

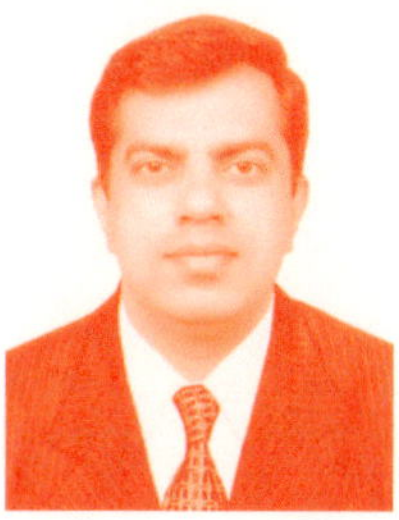
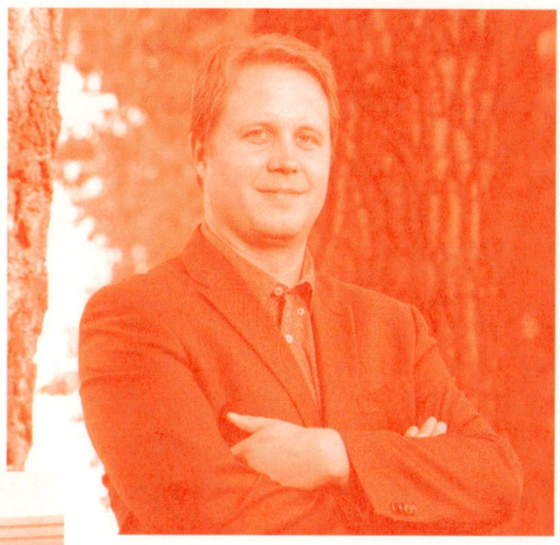
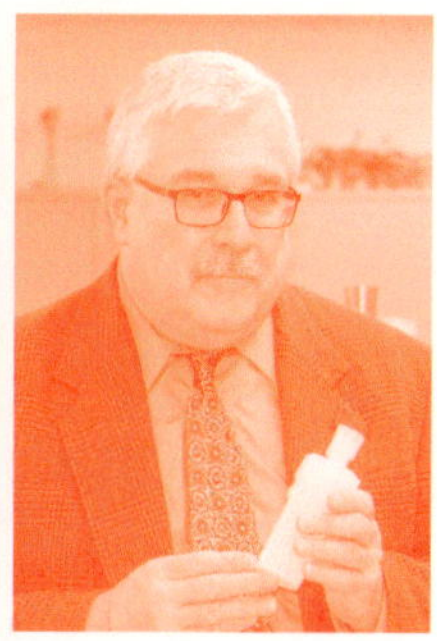
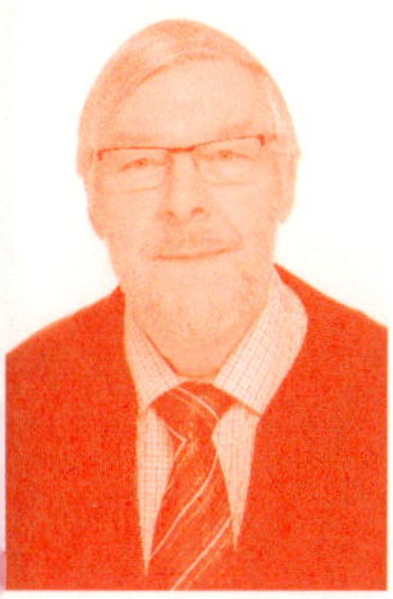
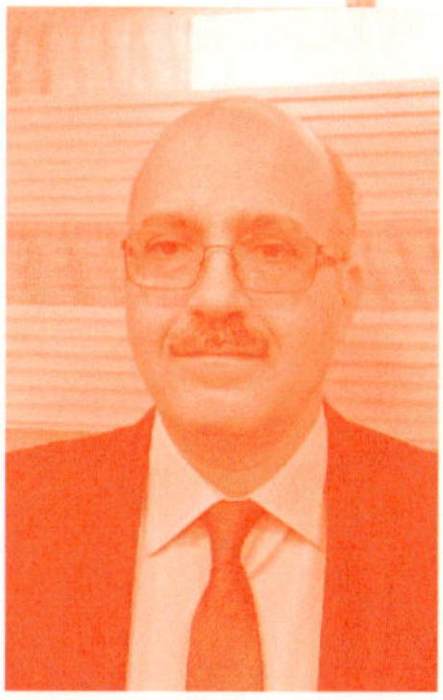
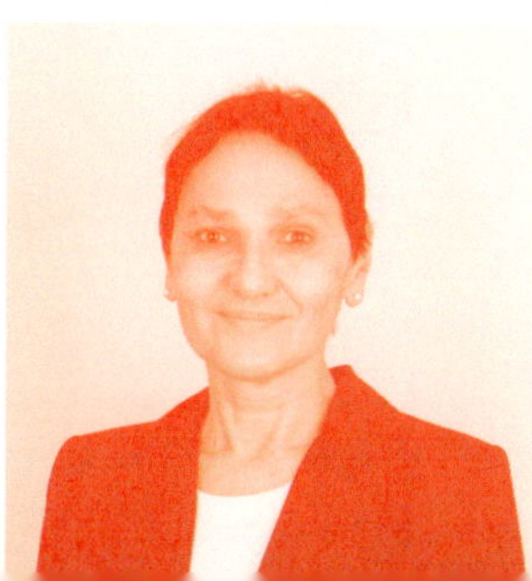
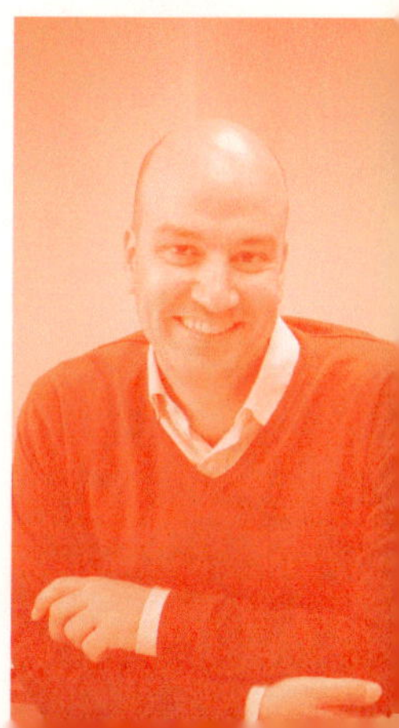

Multidisciplinary Approach for Colorectal Cancer
http://dx.doi.org/10.5772/intechopen.77793
Edited by Keun-Yeong Jeong

Contributors
Susanna Maria Kassier, Heidi Abrahamse, Cherie Kruger, Lenuce Ribeiro Aziz Ydy, Willian Ricardo Camarço-Silva, Wilson Vilela Medeiros-Filho, Aneta Zygulska, Sandra F. Martins, Filipa Macedo, Nuno Bonito, Adhemar Longatto-Filho, Keun-Yeong Jeong

First published in London, United Kingdom, 2019 by IntechOpen
IntechOpen is the global imprint of INTECHOPEN LIMITED, registered in England and Wales, registration number: 11086078, 7th floor, 10 Lower Thames Street, London, EC3R 6AF, United Kingdom
Printed in Croatia

British Library Cataloguing-in-Publication Data
A catalogue record for this book is available from the British Library

Additional hard and PDF copies can be obtained from orders@intechopen.com

Multidisciplinary Approach for Colorectal Cancer
Edited by Keun-Yeong Jeong
p. cm.
Print ISBN 978-1-78984-399-6
Online ISBN 978-1-78984-400-9
eBook (PDF) ISBN 978-1-83968-043-4

For EU product safety concerns:
IN TECH d.o.o., Prolaz Marije Krucifikse Kozulić 3, 51000 Rijeka, Croatia, info@intechopen.com or visit our website at intechopen.com.

Meet the editor

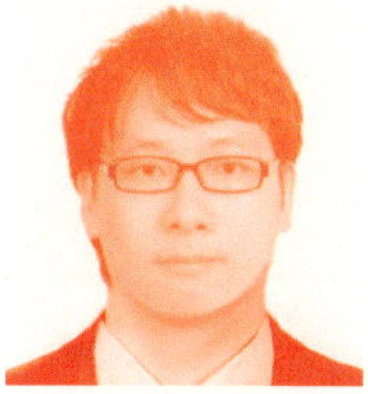

Keun-Yeong Jeong serves as Chief Scientific Officer and Senior Vice President of MetiMedi Pharmaceuticals. Prior to founding MetiMedi Pharmaceuticals, Dr. Jeong focused on investigating cancer. He has noticeable scientific achievements including many peer-reviewed publications and patents. He is also an editor of internationally prominent science journals. Dr. Jeong developed promotion methods for cancer treatment using mesenchymal stem cells and radiation. He received his MS and PhD in Medicine from Korea University, and completed his postdoctoral fellowship at the Yonsei University Cancer Center.

Contents

Preface

Since the importance of the various intracellular environmental changes experienced during the carcinogenesis of colorectal cancer cannot be overlooked, a variety of strategies should be considered. This book describes and examines these strategies.

Chapter 1 provides an introduction and overview of the topics covered herein. Chapter 2 focuses on prevention of colorectal cancer and provides information regarding the role of diet, alcoholic beverages, vitamins, fatness, physical activity, and dietary supplements. Chapter 3 explains the pathogenesis of colorectal cancer as well as examines development of new drugs targeting the disease. Chapter 4 introduces an unconventional method of colorectal cancer therapy, photodynamic therapy, and examines its efficacy. Chapter 5 describes the relationship between immune scores and microbiomes in colorectal cancer prognosis by using a scoring system that analyzes the consequences of the immune balance. The final chapter compares currently available systemic treatment options, efficacy, and safety profiles for understanding patients with advanced colorectal cancer.

The existing colorectal cancer therapies, including surgery, chemotherapy, and radiotherapy, are indispensable options, however, there is plenty of room for improvement in efficacy and toxicity. And the process for these improvements is always in progress. Cancer treatment is expected to be sufficiently improved by adopting a multidisciplinary approach within an integrated framework including initiation, promotion, and progression, under the context of emphasizing the use of standard therapies according to current criteria. In this regard, *Multidisciplinary Approach for Colorectal Cancer* provides useful information for healthcare practitioners and other interested readers.

Keun-Yeong Jeong
Metimedi Pharmaceuticals Co., LTD.,
Senior Vice President,
Head of Research center,
Geobukgol-ro, Seoul,
Republic of Korea

Section 1

Introduction

Chapter 1

Introductory Chapter: Multidisciplinary Colorectal Cancer - First Steps to Encompass Various Strategies for Preventing and Treating Colorectal Cancer

Keun-Yeong Jeong

1. General facts on colorectal cancer

Over the past decades, significant progress has been made in clinical and preclinical sciences. It has been lucky to see the integration of multiple discovery disciplines in science and medicine to push the limits of diagnosis and treatment of disorders that can affect many diseases. However, cancer is an exceptional disease that is relatively intractable and despite the multiple discovery disciplines scholarly. Colorectal cancer (CRC) is the third most common cause of cancer-associated mortality worldwide. According to the data from the National Center for Health Statistics, about 135,000 people are estimated to undergo chemotherapy with CRC in the USA each year, and approximately 50,000 people succumb to the disease annually [1]. Additionally, estimation of the Global Cancer Control project indicated that nearly 2 million people worldwide were diagnosed every year [2]. Well-known option targeting CRC treatment is currently suggested surgical resection preferentially, and if the tumor progression is in an advanced stage, it does require combination with chemotherapy and/or radiation therapy. There is no doubt that surgery, chemotherapy, and radiation therapy are the best choices for treating CRC, even therapeutic efficiency is improving. However, it is still insufficient to reach a convincing level except for the case of early detection; therefore the craving for better potential therapies is still ongoing.

2. Importance of a multidisciplinary approach targeting CRC

To date, the multidisciplinary approach, including initiation, promotion, and progression, which is the process leading to the final diagnosis of CRC is growing interest [3, 4]. These three series of processes belong to carcinogenesis, and it is defined as the process by which environmental and genetic change from normal cells to the final diagnosis of cancer. Initiation includes genetic changes that occur spontaneously or are induced by exposure to carcinogens. Abnormal genetic changes can lead to dysregulation of signaling pathways associated with cell growth, survival, and differentiation [3, 4]. The promotion stage is taken into account in a relatively long and reversible process in which actively growing tumor cells are accumulated. This process is still defined as benign tumor [3, 4]. Progression is a precancerous lesion, before the onset of invasive cancer. It is the last stage of tumor transformation, where genetic and phenotypic changes and cell proliferation occur. This includes a rapid increase in tumor size, and the cells may undergo additional mutations in order to be characterized by invasive and potentially metastatic [3, 4]. As a result of these processes, CRC is finally diagnosed, and after diagnosis, a difficult fight against CRC begins. Therefore, the importance of the various intracellular environmental changes that can be experienced during these three steps of carcinogenesis cannot be overlooked; further, it would encompass the various strategies that can be considered from prevention to treatment targeting CRC pathogenesis and progression. In other words, since the clear concept of effective treatment with less toxicity, which all researchers recognize as important, cannot be convinced by any theory so far, it needs to try a way to share multidisciplinary approaches with many scholars in different disciplines.

3. Multidisciplinary CRC: introduce for contents

In the clinical sense, a multidisciplinary approach for treating CRC means that can support the providing seamless coordination of treatment and has important goals in achieving improved outcomes crucially [5]. As it can be inferred from the foregoing paragraph, however, this book is not intended to emphasize an integrated approach that takes advantage of the optimal options for CRC treatment, including surgery, chemotherapy, and radiation therapy. It contains a variety of unique academic texts on the prevention, prognostic, and therapeutic application for understanding the pathogenesis and progression of CRC. For providing preventative or prolific factors, one chapter provides an overview regarding the role of diet, alcoholic beverages, vitamins, fatness, physical activity, and dietary supplements. Another chapter explains the pathogenesis of CRC, which can be identified as the recent advances in molecular biology, through the risk factors, and also contains contents providing the applicability to new drug development for targeting advanced CRC. In addition, a chapter for therapeutics introduces a method with photodynamic therapy, describing the introduction of unconventional CRC therapy and known efficacy and potential for recent developments. Another chapter includes an introduction to the relationship between immune scores and microbiomes in prognosis in CRC patients by using a scoring system that analyzes the consequences of the immune balance beyond the concept of prognostic prediction through biological markers. In the other chapter, a comparison was made in terms of currently available systemic treatment options, efficacy, and safety profiles for understanding the patients with advanced metastatic colorectal cancer that has remained a challenge for oncologists.

4. Closing remarks

Conventional methods for treating CRC are an indispensable option; however there is enough room for improvement, and related process is always ongoing. This can be overcome by accepting a multidisciplinary concept with unconventional meaning and must be considered in an integrated framework from carcinogenesis, including initiation, promotion, and progression, to final diagnosis, treatment, and prognosis, rather than the significance of the treatment after definite diagnosis. In this regard, the book provides useful information defined "Multidisciplinary Colorectal Cancer."

Conflict of interest

No conflict of interests exists with the publication of this chapter.

Author details

Keun-Yeong Jeong
Metimedi Pharmaceuticals, Republic of Korea

*Address all correspondence to: alvirus@naver.com

References

[1] Siegel RL, Miller KD, Fedewa SA, Ahnen DJ, Meester RGS, Barzi A, et al. Colorectal cancer statistics, 2017. CA: a Cancer Journal for Clinicians. 2017;**67**:177-193. DOI: 10.3322/caac.21395

[2] Bray F, Ferlay J, Soerjomataram I, Siegel RL, Torre LA, Jemal A. Global cancer statistics 2018: GLOBOCAN estimates of incidence and mortality worldwide for 36 cancers in 185 countries. CA: A Cancer Journal for Clinicians. 2018;**68**:394-424. DOI: 10.3322/caac.21492

[3] Siddiqui IA, Sanna V, Ahmad N, Sechi M, Mukhtar H. Resveratrol nanoformulation for cancer prevention and therapy. Annals of the New York Academy of Sciences. 2015;**1348**:20-31. DOI: 10.1111/nyas.12811

[4] Tariq K, Ghias K. Colorectal cancer carcinogenesis: A review of mechanisms. Cancer Biol Med. 2016;**13**:120-35. DOI: 10.28092/j.issn.2095-3941.2015.0103

[5] Augestad KM, Lindsetmo RO, Stulberg J, Reynolds H, Senagore A, Champagne B, et al. International preoperative rectal cancer management: Staging, neoadjuvant treatment, and impact of multidisciplinary teams. World Journal of Surgery. 2010;**34**: 2689-2700. DOI: 10.1007/s00268-010-0738-3

Section 2

Key Factors for Colorectal Cancer Prevention

Chapter 2

Effectivity and Modulating Pathways for the Prevention of Colorectal Cancer: Diet, Body Fatness, Physical Activity, and Supplementation

Susanna Maria Kassier

Abstract

The global prevalence of colorectal cancer (CRC) is currently the highest in high-income countries. However, a rapid increase in prevalence is starting to emerge in many low-income and middle-income countries. This phenomenon is thought to be related to the adoption of a Western lifestyle, characterized by a lack of physical activity, the consumption of refined cereals, as well as highly processed foods. Other characteristics include a reduction in fruit and vegetable intake with a concomitant increase in the consumption of foods that are energy dense, but lacking in micronutrients. Coupled to the above dietary and lifestyle changes is the advent of an increased prevalence of body fatness and central obesity, as well as a dietary intake that lends itself to increasing the risk of developing CRC. As there are observed inconsistencies when appraising the effectivity of dietary and lifestyle-cancer relationships, this chapter will provide an overview of the current body of evidence regarding the role of diet and proxies for lifestyle in terms of their preventative or causative roles in the development of CRC. In addition, the strength of scientific evidence will be alluded to, as well as the modulating pathways responsible for CRC causation or protection.

Keywords: alcohol, body fatness, colorectal cancer, dairy products, diet, dietary fiber, fruits, vegetables, physical activity, processed meat, red meat, supplements

1. Introduction

Globally, colorectal cancer (CRC) is the third most commonly diagnosed malignancy and the fourth leading cause of cancer-related mortality, accounting for about 1.4 million new cases and almost 700,000 deaths in 2012 [1]. Its disease burden is expected to increase by 60%, resulting in over 2.2 million new cases and 1.1 million cancer deaths by 2030 [2]. The distribution of CRC burden varies widely across regions, as more than two-thirds of all cases and about 60% of all deaths occur in countries with a high or very high Human Development Index [1]. However, CRC is considered to be one of the strongest indicators of the global cancer transition, as countries undergoing rapid social and economic transition are displaying rapid increases in the prevalence of cancers that are already more widespread in high-income countries [2]. Hence, CRC incidence and mortality rates are still rapidly increasing in many low-income and middle-income countries, while stabilizing or decreasing trends are being observed in highly developed countries where rates remain among the highest in the world [2]. As patterns and trends in CRC incidence and mortality are related to development levels, their incremental changes could be indicative of the adoption of a more Westernized lifestyle [2].

Targeted interventions tailored to available resources, including primary prevention, are necessary to decrease the global prevalence of CRC [2], as primary prevention dietary habits and other healthy lifestyle factors such as physical activity (PA) are viewed as the most effective and affordable strategy for curbing this global epidemic [3, 4]. In addition, genetic predisposition and environmental factors including diet and PA are considered to be the two main causes of CRC [3, 5].

Due to observed inconsistencies when appraising the effectivity of dietary and lifestyle-cancer relationships, this chapter will provide an overview of the current body of evidence regarding the role of diet, individual foods, alcoholic beverages, vitamins, body fatness, physical activity, and dietary supplements in terms of their classification as preventative or causative in the development of CRC. In addition, the strength of scientific evidence will be alluded to, as well as the modulating pathways responsible for reaping protective benefits or promoting carcinogenesis. Inconsistent findings across scientific literature related to dietary prevention of CRC include but are not limited to discrepancies in study design, dietary interventions assessed, baseline eating patterns, and populations sampled [6].

2. Diet

2.1 Dietary fiber

Dietary fiber refers to carbohydrate polymers of plant origin that may or may not be associated to plant lignin [7]. There is convincing evidence that consuming wholegrains and foods containing dietary fiber decrease the risk of developing CRC [8]. A meta-analysis of prospective studies noted a 10% reduction in CRC risk for every 10 g of total dietary fiber consumed on a daily basis [9]. An analysis of specific sources of dietary fiber found that cereal fiber was associated with a dose-dependent reduction in risk of 10% for every 10 g consumed; however, fruit fibers, vegetable fibers, and legume fibers were not associated with a significant reduction in risk. A meta-analysis of case-control studies and cohort studies on dietary fiber intake and the incidence of CRC adenoma reported similar findings [10].

The European Prospective Investigation into Cancer and Nutrition (EPIC) supports the protective effect of dietary fiber, as the consumption of cereal fiber was significantly and inversely associated with colorectal cancer, colon cancer, and rectal cancer [11]. A significant inverse association was also noted between colon cancer and combined fruit and vegetable fiber intake, although the study was limited by dietary intake assessment conducted at baseline [12].

The HELGA prospective study agrees with previous studies, as a 26% reduction in colon cancer risk in men was reported for every 10 g of dietary fiber consumed on a daily basis. However, the association was not significant in women, thereby suggesting that dietary fiber may be protective against CRC, but other factors such as phytochemicals, energy intake, body weight, and genetics may be equally influential, as is general dietary pattern [13]. This finding serves to demonstrate that consuming dietary fiber from a variety of sources (cereals, fruits, and vegetables) protects against the development of CRC in a dose-dependent manner. Based on the convincing evidence available, it would be reasonable to recommend an increased intake of wholegrains to help reduce the risk of CRC [4].

2.1.1 Mechanism

Dietary fiber found in wholegrains may protect against the development of CRC by increasing fecal bulk through binding water and decreasing colonic transit time, thereby reducing the potential for fecal mutagens to interact with the colon mucosa, lowering the concentration of potential carcinogens, and exposing the colon mucosa to potential carcinogens for shorter period of time [4, 12, 14–17]. In addition, dietary fiber is fermented by intestinal microbiota into short-chain fatty acids (SCFAs) such as butyrate, which in experimental studies was shown to have antiproliferative and pro-apoptosis properties [4, 14–18]. SCFAs also lower fecal pH in the colon, thus providing a healthy intestinal environment [18], as well as inhibit chronic inflammation and cancer cell migration/invasion in the colon. However, these activities are only effective within certain physiological concentration ranges of SCFAs [18].

Other mechanisms include a reduction in secondary bile acid production [14], as well as enhancing the health of colonocytes [12] by modifying the composition of gut microbiota that can enhance immunity [18]. High-fiber diets may also reduce insulin resistance, a risk factor for CRC [7, 8, 14–16], by decreasing insulin growth factor (IGF)-1 activity, decreasing systemic inflammation via the production of SCFAs, and enhancing levels of colonic microbiota, thereby strengthening the intestinal barrier [4, 15, 16]. The anticarcinogenic properties of wholegrains also include being a source of antioxidants such as vitamin E, selenium, copper, zinc, and phytochemicals, as well as decreasing body adiposity [4, 14]. Wholegrains are also sources of lignans, phytoestrogens, and phenolic compounds [14], with many of these bioactive compounds being largely found in the bran and germ of the grain. To illustrate the plausible anticarcinogenic properties of several phenolic acids, experimental studies have showcased their ability to stimulate anti-oxidative activity [19].

2.2 Dairy products

Dairy products include milk (whole or skim milk), cheese (fresh, cottage, and hard cheese), and yogurt [17]. There is strong probable evidence that consuming dairy products, i.e., total dairy, milk, cheese, and dietary calcium, decreases the risk of CRC [8]. Dose-response meta-analyses of dairy products, milk, and dietary calcium were statistically significant with little or no heterogeneity. However, the evidence for cheese was not as strong as for other dairy products, with prospective studies finding no association between cheese intake and CRC risk, thus qualifying the level of evidence as not conclusive [7]. A pooled analysis reported significant inverse associations when comparing the highest with the lowest levels of milk intake and dietary calcium. Hence, there is evidence of plausible mechanisms in humans [8]. As there is probable evidence that milk consumption protects against CRC, it may be reasonable to encourage the consumption of milk for the prevention of CRC [4].

2.2.1 Mechanism

Dairy products contain a variety of bioactive compounds that could be related to simultaneous positive or negative effects on carcinogenesis. The overriding theory underpinning the possible protective effect of dairy products against cancer risk is related to their calcium and to a lesser extent, their vitamin D, lactoferrin, and fermentation products [4, 20, 21]. In addition, dairy products have the ability to modulate inflammatory responses [22]. Lactic acid-producing bacteria may also protect against CRC [20], while the casein and lactose in milk may increase calcium bioavailability [4, 23]. Lastly, the anticarcinogenic effect of milk is also related to its conjugated linoleic acid and butyric acid content [4].

2.3 Red meat

There is strong probable evidence from epidemiologic studies that the consumption of red meat, including beef, pork, lamb, and goat from domesticated animals, increases the risk for developing CRC [7, 8]. The evidence for red meat has consistently shown a positive association in the dose-response meta-analyses for colorectal, colon, and rectal cancer. Despite the result being positive, it was not significant for colorectal and rectal cancers but significant for colon cancer. As there is evidence of plausible mechanisms operating in humans, the consumption of red meat is probably a cause of CRC [8]. In contrast to red meat, the consumption of poultry and fish has been associated with a modest reduction in CRC incidence. This is concordant with the concept that there are components other than fat and protein in red and processed meat that contribute to carcinogenic effects. Thus, based on current evidence, it would be reasonable to recommend the substitution of red and processed meat with poultry or fish, as it can serve as a strategy for CRC prevention [4].

2.3.1 Mechanism

Red meat consists of compounds such as haem iron (HI) that facilitates the endogenous formation of N-nitroso compounds (NOCs) such as nitrosylated HI, catalyzing its formation from natural precursors in the gastrointestinal tract (GI), as well as through lipid peroxidation in the GI [4, 24, 25]. In addition, HI can induce oxidative stress, colonocyte proliferation through the lipid-peroxidation pathway, and production of free radicals in the colonic stream [25]. The carcinogenic compounds forming during processing and cooking include NOCs and polycyclic aromatic hydrocarbons (PAHs) [25]. Cooking red or processed meat at high temperatures produces mutagens such as PAHs and heterocyclic aromatic amine (HAAs) [4, 25], both of which have been linked to CRC development in experimental studies [26]. The latter are genotoxic, and the extent to which HAAs' conversion to genotoxic metabolites occurs as a result of amino acids and creatinine reacting at high cooking temperatures is higher in humans than experimental animals. HAAs become DNA-alkylating agents, inducing DNA mutations after activation by various metabolizing enzymes. The GI microbiota adapts to meat intake and HAAs, resulting in HAAs possibly becoming more genotoxic in those with a high meat intake. However, the majority of studies that have investigated meat and phenotype interactions did not yield convincing evidence. It is therefore probable though that heat-induced mutagens found on the surface of well-done red meat can cause colon cancer in those with a genetic predisposition. NOCs, PAHs, and HAAs are considered to be genotoxic by acting directly on DNA, causing point mutations, deletions, and insertions. However, there is little direct evidence that these mechanisms come into play following meat consumption. A high consumption of HI (excluding other forms of iron), NOCs, HAAs, and PAHs has been associated with an increased risk of colorectal tumors, with a few exceptions. Genetic variations in NOCs' and HAAs' metabolism may alter the relationship between the consumption of red meat and the risk of developing colon cancer. However, there is substantial supporting mechanistic evidence regarding HI, NOCs, and HAAs being involved in colon carcinogenesis. A high consumption of red meat (300–420 g/day), increased levels of DNA adducts, is presumed to be derived from NOCs, in exfoliated colonocytes or rectal biopsies [25].

2.4 Processed meat

There is strong convincing evidence that consuming processed meat, i.e., meats preserved by smoking, curing, or salting, or addition of chemical preservatives, increases the risk of CRC [7, 8]. The evidence is generally consistent by showing an increased risk of CRC with increased consumption of processed meat. The dose-response meta-analysis showed a significant increased risk of CRC at consumption levels of 50 g/day [8].

2.4.1 Mechanism

The carcinogenic compounds that form during processing include NOCs and PAHs. NOCs are exogenously introduced from nitrates and nitrites added during the preservation process [25, 27] but can also be formed endogenously. In processed meat, HI is nitrosylated because curing salt contains nitrate or nitrite. There is evidence that nitrosylated HI promotes carcinogenesis at doses that are five to six times lower than non-nitrosylated HI [25].

However, it is likely that a combination of mechanisms contribute to a higher risk of developing CRC among those who consume high quantities of processed meat. Similar to red meat, processed meat is high in fat, protein, and HI, which can promote carcinogenesis through the mechanisms described under red meat [25, 26]. In addition, processed meats such as sausages are often cooked at high temperatures, leading to increased exposure to HAAs and PAHs [25, 27], with levels varying according to meat type, temperature, cooking time, and method [25]. The invariably higher fat content of processed meat when compared to red meat may stimulate carcinogenesis through synthesis of secondary bile acids. However, human data supporting this hypothesis are weak [27].

2.5 Fruits

A dose-response meta-analysis showed no significant association between fruit consumption and CRC. There was evidence of a nonlinear dose response of CRC and fruit intake showing a significant increased risk at low levels (less than 100 g per day) of intake [7, 8]. Hence there is limited suggestive evidence available that a low consumption of fruit increases the risk of colorectal [8].

2.5.1 Mechanism

Apart from fiber content, fruits are a rich source of vitamins C and E, as well as numerous bioactive compounds which may have an anticarcinogenic potential. These include folate, flavonoids, polyphenols, and limonene [4, 28]. Many of these compounds have potent anti-oxidative properties which could inhibit cellular damage and exposure to reactive oxygen species [28].

2.6 Non-starchy vegetables

Based on epidemiological studies, the term vegetables may cover different categories, namely, total vegetables (non-starchy vegetables and starchy vegetables), non-starchy vegetables, fresh vegetables (as opposed to preserved vegetables), and raw vegetables (excluding cooked vegetables) [7]. There is limited suggestive evidence that a low intake (less than 100 g per day) of cruciferous vegetables and non-starchy vegetables might increase the risk of CRC [7, 8]. However, there is also limited evidence that a high intake of fruits and vegetables protects against

CRC. Considering the well-establish cardiometabolic benefits of adequate fruit and vegetable intake, it would be reasonable to recommend increasing intake among populations with very low consumption [4].

2.6.1 Mechanism

The consumption of vegetables provides a large number of potential anticarcinogenic components that include dietary fiber, carotenoids, vitamins C and E, selenium, folate, dithiolethiones, glucosinolates and indoles, isothiocyanates, flavonoids, polyphenols, protease inhibitors, plant sterols, allium compounds, and limonene [7, 29]. It is possible that a combination of these nutrients and phytochemicals is responsible for the lower CRC risks associated with vegetable consumption [8], due to their antioxidant and antiproliferative activities, modulating xenobiotic and hormonal metabolism and immunity [30, 31]. Vegetables are an important source of micronutrients, notably folate that plays an important role in DNA synthesis and methylation and in the expression of genes involved in carcinogenesis [32]. Anticarcinogenic compounds such as folate, vitamins, fiber, minerals, flavonoids, and glucosinolates are found in cruciferous vegetables [4].

2.7 Alcoholic beverages

Alcoholic beverages contain ethanol that is formed during fermentation. In epidemiological studies, exposure to alcoholic beverages is examined by measures such as drinking or not, the number of drinks/glasses or 10 g units consumed per day or per week [7]. Concerning CRC associations, the evidence is considered to be convincing in men and probable in women [7, 33], as there is convincing evidence that the consumption of approximately two or more alcoholic drinks per day (30 g) increases the risk of CRC with a significant risk being observed for colorectal, colon, and rectal cancer [8]. An intake of 30 g per day is associated with a 16% increase in CRC risk, whereas an intake of 45 g per day increases the risk by 41% [34], suggesting a dose-response relationship in which the higher the intake, the higher the risk [33].

2.7.1 Mechanism

The mechanisms whereby chronic alcohol consumption has an effect on the development of CRC are diverse. Acetaldehyde (the first compound formed in ethanol metabolism) has mutagenic and carcinogenic activity. It is thought that it plays a critical role in CRC onset via toxic metabolites of ethanol oxidation that can be carcinogenic to colonocytes [35, 36]. Higher ethanol consumption can also induce oxidative stress through the increased production of reactive oxygen species which are genotoxic and carcinogenic [37]. Alcohol may also act as a solvent for cellular penetration of dietary or environmental (e.g., tobacco) carcinogens, affect hormone metabolism, and interfere with retinoid metabolism and with DNA repair mechanisms [38].

3. Vitamins

3.1 Vitamin C

There is limited suggestive evidence that consuming foods containing vitamin C might decrease the risk of colon cancer. However, no conclusion was drawn regarding rectal cancer [8]. Although the evidence was limited, it was generally consistent and the dose-response meta-analysis showed a significant decreased risk at a level of 40 mg per day [8].

3.1.1 Mechanism

The biological plausibility to support a protective effect of vitamin C on CRC development is related to its potency as an antioxidant, thereby reducing levels of reactive oxygen species, inhibiting lipid peroxidation, and reducing nitrates [4, 28]. Vitamin C has also been shown to inhibit carcinogen formation in experimental models and to protect DNA from mutagenic effects [39]. Other mechanisms include inhibition of cell proliferation, pro-apoptosis, and a reduction in inflammation [4].

3.2 Vitamin D

There is limited suggestive evidence that foods containing vitamin D, serum vitamin D, and supplemental vitamin D might decrease the risk of CRC [8]. For foods containing vitamin D, a dose-response meta-analysis showed a significant decreased risk for CRC. For supplemental vitamin D, the dose-response meta-analysis showed a significant decreased risk for colon cancer, whereas for plasma/serum vitamin D, the dose-response meta-analysis did not exhibit a significant association with CRC. Two published meta-analyses reported significant inverse associations. Hence, the WCRF/AICR, Continuous Update Project report, noted that plasma/serum vitamin D status can be influenced by sun exposure, obesity, seasonality, smoking, and measurement error. There is evidence of plausible mechanisms in humans [8]. Convincing data from epidemiologic and experimental studies support the potential chemopreventive effects of vitamin D against CRC development, although the evidence from randomized controlled trials (RCTs) is inconclusive [4].

3.2.1 Mechanism

Underlying mechanisms for an effect of vitamin D on CRC have been predominantly studied in vitro and experimental models. Hence, limited data is available in humans [8]. However, these studies suggest a role of circulating vitamin D through its active form, 1 α, 12-dihydroxyvitamin D3 [1,12(OH)2D3], in controlling cell growth, by reducing proliferation and by inducing differentiation and apoptosis [4, 40]. Other alleged mechanisms related to a higher vitamin D status are related to improved innate and adaptive immune function, inhibition of angiogenesis, reduced inflammation, and regulation of microRNA expression [4, 40–42], as well as inhibition of invasion and metastasis and suppression of angiogenesis [4].

4. Body fatness

Body fatness and abdominal obesity is normally estimated by body mass index (BMI), waist circumference, and waist-to-hip ratio [7]. There is strong convincing evidence that body fatness increases the risk of colorectal, colon, and rectum cancer [7]. However, cognizance should be taken of the fact that these anthropometric measurements have limitations as they do not distinguish between lean and fat mass [8]. Evidence supporting a clear dose-response association was related to showing a significant increased risk of CRC with an increased BMI [8, 43, 44]. There is evidence of a nonlinear dose response, whereby the increased risk is higher at a BMI beyond 27 kg/m^2 for CRC. Significant positive associations were observed for CRC in the dose-response analysis for waist circumference and waist-to-hip ratio [8]; hence, the level of evidence is being referred to as convincing for abdominal obesity [33]. In contrast to the vague findings regarding the role of individual nutrients or foods, the strong consistent association between obesity and CRC (at least in men) further underscores the importance of combined integrated effects of nutrients/foods over their individual effects. These effects probably do not only reflect the imbalance between energy intake and expenditure but the often suboptimal quality of the diet associated with the development of obesity [4].

4.1 Mechanism

Overnutrition increases the supply of glucose and fat that can feed into metabolic reprogramming to fuel cancer cell proliferation. In addition, glycolysis has been shown to be enhanced in cancer cells of obese individuals. As obesity is often associated with metabolic syndrome (MS) and diabetes, characterized by hyperglycemia and/or hypertriglyceridemia, an abundance of circulating nutrients are available for tumor development, even between feeding periods [45]. Autophagy, the process whereby cancer cells digest and recycle their cellular contents during periods of low nutrient availability, can provide cancer cells with lipids, amino acids, and nucleotides required for proliferation [46]. Obesity has been shown to induce autophagy, particularly in adipocytes [45]. These obesity-associated metabolic adaptations facilitate the development of cancer traits that include insensitivity to anti-growth signals, resistance to cell death, and deregulation of cellular energetics [47]. Hence, interactions between cancer cell energetics and systemic metabolism highlight unique therapeutic strategies and interventions, particularly among obese individuals, as cancer cells may be more sensitive to metabolic interference, having already committed to metabolic reprogramming [45].

In addition, obesity and MS are associated with abnormalities in insulin signaling, growth factor signaling, and glucose metabolism [48]. One growth factor implicated in cancer risk and progression is insulin-like growth factor (IGF)-1. Hyperglycemia and hyperinsulinemia, diagnostic criteria of MS, increase IGF-1 production and bioavailability. Furthermore, hyperglycemia suppresses IGF-1-binding protein synthesis, while hyperinsulinemia promotes expression of growth hormone receptor and subsequent IGF-1 synthesis [48]. Growth and survival functions of IGF-1 give it the potential to have an impact on many characteristics of cancer, including sustained proliferative signaling, insensitivity to anti-growth signals, induction of angiogenesis, and metastatic potential [49]. As a result, elevated IGF-1 has been established as a risk factor for CRC [45].

Higher body fatness is associated with increased insulin levels, which can promote cell growth and inhibit apoptosis and has been linked to a greater risk of CRC in humans [50, 51] and in experimental studies [52]. Body fatness also stimulates the body's inflammatory response, which can promote CRC development [53, 54]. Overall, there are convincing mechanistic data supporting a link between body fatness and CRC [8].

5. Physical activity

Physical activity (PA) includes all movements performed in daily life, including sport, whether recreational or competitive [30], as well as that performed in occupational, transport, recreational, and household settings [7]. In epidemiological studies, PA is computed by combining intensity, duration, and frequency of different types of PA, with subjects being classified into three levels of PA, namely, low, moderate, or high. PA is usually divided into four types of activity related to occupational, transport, recreational, and household settings. Total PA is calculated as the sum of the four types or any of the four types that are presented as all-type PA. Thus a major barrier to conducting meta-analyses is the disparity between the measures of PA [7].

There is convincing evidence that all types of PA, when comparing the highest and lowest levels, are protective against colon cancer with a significant inverse association being observed for total PA and CRC. However, no significant associations were observed for rectal cancer and either total or recreational PA when comparing the highest and lowest levels. For recreational PA and colon cancer risk, three published meta-analysis reported inverse associations. In addition, there is robust evidence for mechanisms operating in humans. However, dose-response relationships could not be determined [7, 8]. The protective effect was similar for proximal and distal colon cancer and was stronger for men than women [7]. More physically active subjects had a 24% decreased risk of CRC compared to those who lead a more sedentary lifestyle [55]. It has been reported that those who exercise regularly decrease their CRC risk by 40%, regardless of BMI [56]. In addition, 30 min of daily moderate exercise result in an 11% reduction in CRC [57].

5.1 Mechanism

PA reduces body fatness and therefore has a beneficial effect on CRC risk, possibly due to a reduction in insulin resistance and inflammation [50, 53, 54]. However, it is unclear whether PA that is not accompanied by weight loss has a significant impact on these pathways. Other mechanisms through which PA may lower CRC risk include the stimulation of digestion and reduction of gastrointestinal (GI) transit time, although robust data to support this mechanism in humans is limited [58]. Overall, mechanistic data to support a link between PA and CRC are moderate in strength [8].

6. Supplementation

6.1 Calcium changes made to this section are indicated in blue

The Women's Health Initiative failed to show a significant relationship between calcium supplementation and the risk of developing CRC among postmenopausal women [59], while a meta-analysis of cohort studies reported a significant inverse relationship for colon and CRC when comparing the highest to lowest levels of calcium supplementation [60]. As there is evidence of plausible mechanisms in humans, the Continuous Update Project (CUP) panel concluded that taking calcium supplements probably protect against CRC, based on evidence derived from a dosage of more than 200 mg per day [8]. The evidence was generally consistent and showed inverse associations across a range of intakes (200–1000 mg). RCTs reported a nonsignificant inverse association for calcium and vitamin D supplementation compared to placebo, after excluding women using calcium or vitamin D supplements at baseline. Although no dose-response meta-analysis could be conducted, six of the eight cohort studies reported inverse associations [8]. Predominant evidence indicates an increased CRC risk among individuals with a calcium intake lower than 700–1000 mg/day. It would therefore be reasonable to encourage individuals to increase their calcium intake to a level above this range, while recognizing that available data yielded inconsistent results [4].

6.1.1 Mechanism

A proposed mechanism for the protective properties of calcium against CRC is its ability to bind to unconjugated bile acids and free fatty acids (FFAs), thereby limiting their toxic effects on the colorectum [4, 61]. Cell culture studies suggest that it may also suppress cell proliferation and promote cell differentiation and apoptosis, likely by influencing different cell-signaling pathways [4, 62]. Calcium may also prevent colonic K-ras mutations and inhibit haem-induced promotion of colon carcinogenesis [63, 64]. In addition, calcium also inhibits oxidative DNA damage and modulates CRC-related cell-signaling pathways [4].

6.2 Multivitamins-multivitamins were kept under the heading of "Supplementation" as the content under "Vitamins" in Section 3 is related to vitamins derived from whole foods and not supplements

There is evidence that consuming multivitamin supplements might decrease the risk of CRC cancer [8]. However, the evidence is limited but generally consistent [8]. One RCT in men reported a nonsignificant inverse association for multivitamin supplementation compared to placebo. The analysis of highest versus lowest users of supplements showed a significant decreased risk of CRC. One published meta-analysis on CRC and colon cancer reported significant inverse associations. There is evidence of plausible mechanisms in humans [8].

6.2.1 Mechanism

Multivitamin supplements consist of a combination of several, or in some instances, many vitamins, thereby making it challenging to determine what exactly the active ingredient is. Numerous vitamins included in multivitamin supplements have been shown to neutralize free radicals and reactive oxygen species and to prevent lipid peroxidation [65].

7. Conclusion

Based on the dietary- and lifestyle-related evidence presented, there is convincing evidence that PA decreases the risk of developing CRC, while the consumption of processed meat increases risk. In addition, the consumption of alcoholic beverages is a convincing cause of CRC, as is higher body fatness. Probable evidence regarding a decreased risk for the development of CRC is available for the consumption of wholegrains, foods containing dietary fiber, dairy products, and calcium supplements. There is also probable evidence that the consumption of red meat probably causes CRC. Limited suggestive evidence regarding the prevention of CRC exists for foods containing vitamin C and vitamin D and taking a multivitamin supplement, while the same level of evidence for increasing CRC risk is related to a low consumption of non-starchy vegetables and fruits.

For the prevention of cancer, it is recommended that the general population should strive toward maintaining a healthy weight, being physically active, eating a variety of foods, and limiting alcohol intake. However, recommendations aimed at the prevention of CRC, include keeping body weight within a healthy range, being physically active, making wholegrains, vegetables, fruit, and legumes a major part of the usual diet, and limiting the consumption of fast foods and other processed foods high in fat, starches, and sugars. Furthermore, red meat should be consumed in moderate amounts, while little if any processed meat should be consumed. It is best not to drink alcohol and not using supplements for the prevention of CRC.

Conflict of interest

The author has no conflict of interest associated with this publication.

Author details

Susanna Maria Kassier
Dietetics and Human Nutrition, College of Agriculture, Engineering and Science, University of KwaZulu-Natal, Pietermaritzburg, South Africa

*Address all correspondence to: kassiers@ukzn.ac.za

References

[1] Ferlay J, Soerjomataram I, Evik M, et al. Cancer incidence and mortality worldwide: Sources, methods and major patterns in GLOBOCAN 2012. International Journal of Cancer. 2015;**136**(5):E359-E386. DOI: 10.1002/ijc.29210

[2] Arnold M, Sierra MS, Laversanne M, et al. Global patterns and trends in colorectal cancer incidence and mortality. Gut. 2017;**66**:683-691. DOI: 10.1136/gutjnl-2015-310912

[3] Boyle P, Leon ME. Epidemiology of colorectal cancer. British Medical Bulletin. 2002;**64**(1):1-25. DOI: 10.1093/bmb/64.1.1

[4] Song M, Garrett WS, Chan AT. Nutrients, foods, and colorectal cancer prevention. Gastroenterology. 2015;**148**:1244-1260. DOI: 10.1053/j.gastro.2014.12.035

[5] Chambers WM, Warren BF, Jewell DT, et al. Cancer surveillance in ulcerative colitis. The British Journal of Surgery. 2005;**92**:928-936. DOI: 10.1002/bjs.5106

[6] Emenaker NJ, Ragas AJ. Nutrition and cancer research: Resources for the nutrition and dietetics practitioner. Journal of the American Dental Association (Chicago, IL). 2017;**118**:550-554. DOI: 10.101/j.jand.2017.10.011

[7] Latino-Martel P, Cottet V, Druesne-Pecollo N, et al. Alcoholic beverages, obesity, physical activity and other nutritional factors, and cancer risk: A review of the evidence. Critical Reviews in Oncology/Hematology. 2016;**99**:303-323. DOI: 10.1016/j.critrevonc.2016.01.002

[8] WCRF/AICR. Continuous Update Project Expert Report. Diet, nutrition, physical activity and colorectal cancer 2018 [Internet]. 2018. Available from: www.wcrf.org/sites/default/files/Dietandcancerreport.org [Accessed: January 01, 2019]

[9] Aune D, Chan DS, Lau R, et al. Dietary fibre, whole grains, and risk of colorectal cancer: Systematic review and dose-response meta-analysis of prospective studies. BMJ. 2011;**343**:d6617. DOI: 10.1136/bmj.d6617

[10] Ben Q, Sun Y, Chai R, et al. Dietary fibre intakes reduces risk for colorectal adenoma: A meta-analysis. Gastroenterology. 2014;**146**(3):689, e6-699. DOI: 10.1053/j.gastro.2013.11.003

[11] Murphy N, Norat T, Ferrari P, et al. Dietary fibre intake and the risks of cancers of the colon and rectum in the European Prospective Investigation into Cancer and Nutrition (EPIC). PLoS One. 2012;**7**(6):e39361. DOI: 10.1371/journal.pone.0039361

[12] Dahl WJ, Stewart ML. Position of the academy of nutrition and dietetics: Health implications of dietary fibre. Journal of the American Dental Association (Chicago, IL). 2015;**115**(11):1861-1870. DOI: 10.1016/j.jand.2015.09.003

[13] Hansen I, Skeie G, Landberg R, et al. Intake of dietary fibre, especially from cereal foods, is associated with lower incidence of colon cancer in the HELGA cohort. International Journal of Cancer. 2012;**131**(2):469-478. DOI: 10.1002/ijc.26381

[14] Slavin J. Fibre and prebiotics: Mechanisms and health benefits. Nutrients. 2013;**5**(4):1417-1435. DOI: 10.3390/nu5041417

[15] Canani RB, Costanzo MD, Leone L, et al. Potential beneficial effects of butyrate in intestinal and

extraintestinal diseases. World Journal of Gastroenterology. 2011;**17**(12): 1519-1528. DOI: 10.3748/wjg.v17.i12.1519

[16] Moore MA, Park CB, Tsuda H. Soluble and insoluble fiber influences on cancer development. Critical Reviews in Oncology/Hematology. 1998;**27**(3):229-242. DOI: 10.1016/S1040-8428(98)00006-7

[17] Kaczmarczyk MM, Miller MJ, Freund GG. The health benefits of dietary fiber: Beyond the usual suspects of type 2 diabetes mellitus, cardiovascular disease and colon cancer. Metabolism. 2012;**61**(8):1058-1066. DOI: 10.1016/j.metabol.2012.01.017

[18] Zeng H, Lazarova DL, Bordonaro M. Mechanisms lining dietary fiber, gut microbiota and colon cancer prevention. World Journal of Gastrointestinal Oncology. 2014;**6**(2):41-51. DOI: 10.4251/wjgo.v6.i2.416

[19] Kim KH, Tsao R, Yang R, et al. Phenolic acid profiles and antioxidant activities of wheat bran extracts and the effect of hydrolysis conditions. Food Chemistry. 2006;**95**:466-473. DOI: 10.1016/j.foodchem.2005.01.032

[20] Norat R, Riboli E. Dairy products and colorectal cancer. A review of possible mechanisms and epidemiologic evidence. European Journal of Clinical Nutrition. 2003;**57**(1):1-17. DOI: 10.1038/sj.ejcn.1601522

[21] Tsuda H, Kozu T, Iinuma G, et al. Cancer prevention by bovine lactoferrin: From animal studies to human trial. BioMetals. 2010;**23**(3):399-409. DOI: 10.1007/s10534-010-9331-3

[22] Bordoni A, Danesi F, Dardevet D, et al. Dairy products and inflammation: A review of the clinical evidence. Critical Reviews in Food Science and Nutrition. 2017;**57**(12):2497-2525. DOI: 10.1080/10408398. 2014.967385

[23] Guengen L, Pointillart A. The bioavailability of dietary calcium. Journal of the American College of Nutrition. 2000;**19**(2 Suppl):119S-136S

[24] Cross AJ, Pollock JR, Bigham SA. Haem, not protein or inorganic iron, is responsible for endogenous intestinal N-nitrosation arising from red meat. Cancer Research. 2003;**63**(10):2358-2360

[25] Kassier SM. Colon cancer and the consumption of red and processed meat: An association that is medium, rare or well done? SAJCN. 2016;**29**(4):145-149. DOI: 1o.1080/16070658.2016.1217645

[26] Cross AJ, Sinha R. Meat-related mutagens/carcinogens in the etiology of colorectal cancer. Environmental and Molecular Mutagenesis. 2004;**44**(1):44-55

[27] Santarelli RL, Pierre F, Corper DE. Processed meat and colorectal cancer: A review of epidemiologic and experimental evidence. Nutrition and Cancer. 2008;**60**:131-144. DOI: 10.1080/01635580701684872

[28] Lü JM, Lin PH, Yao Q, et al. Chemical and molecular mechanisms of antioxidants: Experimental approaches and model systems. Journal of Cellular and Molecular Medicine. 2010;**14**:840-860. DOI: 10.1111/j.1582-4934.2009.00897

[29] Steinmetz KA, Potter JD. Vegetables, fruit, and cancer. II. Mechanisms. Cancer Causes & Control. 1991;**2**:427-442

[30] WHO. Global Recommendations on Physical Activity for Health [Internet]. Available from: http://apps.who.int/iris/bitstream/10665/44399/1/9789241599979.eng.pdf [Accessed: January 01, 2019]

[31] Liu J, Wang J, Leng Y, et al. Intake of fruit and vegetables and risk of esophageal

squamous cell carcinoma: A meta-analysis of observational studies. International Journal of Cancer. 2013;**133**(2):473-485. DOI: 10.1002/ijc.28024

[32] Liu B, Mao Q, Lin Y, et al. The association of cruciferous vegetable intake and risk of bladder cancer: A meta-analysis. World Journal of Urology. 2013;**31**(1):127-133. DOI: 10.1007/s00345-012-0850-0

[33] Baena R, Salinas P. Diet and colorectal. Maturitas. 2015;**80**:258-264. DOI: 10.1016/j.maturitas.2014.12.017

[34] Durko L, Malecka-Panas E. Lifestyle modifications colorectal cancer. Current Colorectal Cancer Reports. 2014;**10**(1):45-54. DOI: 10.1007/s11888-013-0203-4

[35] Seitz HK, Stickel F. Molecular mechanisms of alcohol-mediated carcinogenesis. Nature Reviews. Cancer. 2007;7:599-612

[36] Reidy J, McHugh E, Stassen LFA. A review of the relationship between alcohol and oral cancer. The Surgeon. 2011;**9**(5):278-283. DOI: 10.1016/j.surge.2011.01.010

[37] Albano E. Alcohol, oxidative stress and free radical damage. The Proceedings of the Nutrition Society. 2006;**65**:278-290

[38] Boffetta P, Hashibe M. Alcohol and cancer. The Lancet Oncology. 2006;7(2):149-156. DOI: 10.1016/s1470-2045 (06)70577-0

[39] Mirvish SS. Effects of vitamins C and E on N-nitroso compound formation, carcinogenesis, and cancer. Cancer. 1986;**58**:1842-1850

[40] Dou R, Ng K, Giovannucci EL, et al. Vitamin D and colorectal cancer: Molecular, epidemiological and clinical evidence. The British Journal of Nutrition. 2016;**115**(9):1643-1660. DOI: 10.1017/s0007114516000696

[41] van Harten-Gerritsen AS, Balvers MGJ, Witkamp RF, et al. Vitamin D, inflammation, and colorectal cancer progression: A review of mechanistic studies and future directions for epidemiological studies. Cancer Epidemiology, Biomarkers and Prevention. 2015;**24**:1820-1828. DOI: 10.1158/1055-9965.EPI-15-0601

[42] Alvarez-Diaz S, Valle N, Ferrer-Mayorga G, et al. MicroRNA-22 is induced by vitamin D and contributes to its antiproliferative, antimigratory and gene regulatory effects in colon cancer cells. Human Molecular Genetics. 2012;**21**(10):2157-2165. DOI: 10.1093/hmg/dds031

[43] Guh DP, Zhang W, Bansback N, et al. The incidence of co-morbidities related to obesity and overweight: A systematic review and meta-analysis. BMC Public Health. 2009;**9**:88. DOI: 10.1186/1471-2458-9-88

[44] Lauby-Secretan B, Scoccianti C, Loomis D, et al. Body fatness and cancer—Viewpoint of the IARC Working Group. NEJM. 2016;**375**(8):794-798. DOI: 10.1056/NEJMsr1606602

[45] Smith LA, O'Flanagan CH, Bowers LW, et al. Translating mechanism-based strategies to break the obesity-cancer link: A narrative review. Journal of the Academy of Nutrition and Dietetics. 2018;**18**(4):652-667. DOI: 10.1016/j.jand.2017.08.112

[46] Kimmelman AC, White E. Autophagy and tumor metabolism. Cell Metabolism. 2017;**25**(5):1037-1043. DOI: 10.1016/j.cmet.2017.04.004

[47] Donohoe CL, Lysaght J, O'Sullivan J, et al. Emerging concepts linking obesity with the hallmarks of cancer. Trends

in Endocrinology and Metabolism. 2017;**28**(1):46-62. DOI: 10.1016/j.tem.2016.08.004

[48] Braun S, Bitton-Worms K, LeRoith D. The link between the metabolic syndrome and cancer. International Journal of Biological Sciences. 2011;7(7):1003-1015

[49] Brahmkhatri VP, Prasanna C, Atreya HS. Insulin-like growth factor system in cancer: Novel targeted therapies. Biomedical Research Institute. 2015:538019. DOI: 10.1155/2015/538019

[50] Murphy N, Cross AJ, Abubakar M, et al. A nested case-control study of metabolically defined body size phenotypes and risk of colorectal cancer in the European Prospective Investigation into Cancer and Nutrition (EPIC). PLoS Medicine. 2016;**13**:e1001988. DOI: 10.1371/journal.pmed.1001988

[51] Jenab B, Riboli E, Cleveland RJ, et al. Serum C-peptide, IGFBP-1 and IGFBP-2 and risk of colon and rectal cancers in the European Prospective Investigation into Cancer and Nutrition. International Journal of Cancer. 2007;**121**(2):368-376

[52] Tran TT, Naigamwalla D, Oprescu AI, et al. Hyperinsulinemia, but not other factors associated with insulin resistance, acutely enhances colorectal epithelial proliferation in vivo. Endocrinology. 2006;**147**(4):1830-1837

[53] Ho GYF, Wang T, Gunter MJ, et al. Adipokines linking obesity with colorectal cancer risk in postmenopausal women. Cancer Research. 2012;**72**(12):3092-3037. DOI: 10.1158/0008-5472.CAN-11-2771

[54] Zhou B, Shu B, Yang J, et al. C-reactive protein, interleukin-6 and the risk of colorectal cancer: A meta-analysis. Cancer Causes & Control. 2014;**25**(10):1397-1405. DOI: 10.1007/s10552-014-0445-8

[55] Wolin KY, Yan Y, Colditz GA, et al. Physical activity and colon cancer prevention: A meta-analysis. British Journal of Cancer. 2009;**100**(4):611-616. DOI: 10.1038/sj.bjc.660417

[56] Tárraga López PJ, Albero JS, Rodríquez-Montes JA. Is it possible to reduce the incident of colorectal cancer by modifying diet and lifestyle? Current Cancer Therapy Reviews. 2013;**9**(3):157163. DOI: 10.2174/15733947 0903140220144227

[57] Perera PS, Thompson RL, Weseman MJ. Recent evidence for colorectal cancer prevention through healthy food, nutrition, and physical activity: Implications for recommendations. Current Nutrition Reports. 2012;**1**(1):44-54

[58] Song BK, Cho KO, Jo Y, et al. Colon transit time according to physical activity level in adults. Journal of Neurogastroenterology and Motility. 2012;**18**(1):64-69. DOI: 10.5056/jnm.2012.18.1.64

[59] Prentice RL, Pettinger MB, Jackson RD, et al. Health risks and benefits from calcium and vitamin D supplementation: Women's Health Initiative clinical trial and cohort study. Osteoporosis International. 2013;**24**(2):567-580. DOI: 10.1007/s00198-012-2224-2

[60] Huncharek M, Muscat J, Kupelnick B. Colorectal cancer risk and dietary intake of calcium, vitamin D, and dairy products: A meta-analysis of 26,335 cases from 60 observational studies. Nutrition and Cancer. 2009;**61**(1):47-69. DOI: 10.1080/01635580802395733

[61] Newmark HL, Wargovich MJ, Bruce WR. Colon cancer and dietary fat, phosphate, and calcium: A hypothesis.

JNCI. 1984;**72**(6):1323-1325. DOI: 10.1093/jnci/72.6.1323

[62] Fediriko V, Bostick RM, Flanders W, et al. Effects of vitamin D and calcium on proliferation and differentiation in normal colon mucosa: A randomized clinical trial. Cancer Epidemiology, Biomarkers and Prevention. 2009;**18**(11):2933-2941. DOI: 10.1158/1055-9965.EPI-09-0239

[63] Lior X, Jacoby RF, Teng BB, et al. K-ras mutations in 1,2-dimethylhydrazine-induced colonic tumors: Effects op supplemental dietary calcium and vitamin D deficiency. Cancer Research. 1991;**51**(16):4305-4309

[64] Pierre FH, Martin OC, Santarelli RL, et al. Calcium and α-tocopherol suppress cured-meat promotion of chemically-induced colon carcinogenesis in rats and reduce associated biomarkers in human volunteers. The American Journal of Clinical Nutrition. 2013;**98**(5): 1255-1262. DOI: 10.3945/ajcn.113.061069

[65] Heine-Bröring RC, Winkels RM, Renkema JM, et al. Dietary supplement use and colon cancer risk: A systematic review and meta-analyses of prospective cohort studies. International Journal of Cancer. 2015;**136**(10):2388-2401. DOI: 10.1002/ijc.29277

Section 3

Pathogenesis of Colorectal Cancer

Chapter 3

A Genetic Perspective on Colorectal Cancer Progression

Lenuce Ribeiro Aziz Ydy, Willian Ricardo Camarço-Silva and Wilson Vilela Medeiros-Filho

Abstract

The colorectal cancer is one of most frequent neoplasia in adult population. Since was described the adenoma-carcinoma sequence for the first time in 1978, the elucidation of the molecular mechanisms involved in the pathogenesis of colorectal cancer became studied. The study of colorectal cancer has been one of the most important elements for understanding the mechanisms involved in the genesis of malignant neoplasms. Several genes, like DCC, APC, p53 were identified as participants of the adenoma-carcinoma. The annexin A1 protein (ANXA1) is related with some types of tumor and its study in colorectal cancer in scientific literature is been done, but discreetly yet. The increasing advancement in molecular biology research have contributes for understanding the carcinogenesis, with the possibility of detecting earlier pre-malignant lesions and a proper diagnosis, more over it allow the development an efficient therapy.

Keywords: colorectal cancer, molecular biology, carcinogenesis

1. Introduction

Colorectal cancer (CCR) is the third most common cancer in men, the second in women and the third most prevalent cause of mortality in the world. It was estimated more than 1.8 million new cases in 2018 according to American Institute for Cancer Research and Continuous Update project panel. It is linked to the transition nutrition to the western lifestyle, consuming processed meat, red meat and alcoholic drinks, greater body fatness and adult height increase the risk of the disease. The incidence of the disease continues to rise especially in low and middle income countries and it is considered one of the clearest markers for rapid societal and economic changes that are associated with cancer development [1].

Genetic knowledge is essential for understanding of carcinogenic colorectal cancer, and can develop strategies for prevention, diagnosis and treatment. A list of genes in which mutations are capable of interfering with both cancer creation and treatment, has grown a lot in recent years, helping to understand risks for cancer formation and identifying several promising therapeutic targets. Today focused on a best treatment, but research on colorectal cancer genetics began with a focus on diagnosis, much of our understanding of pathogenesis came from study of hereditary syndromes of colorectal diseases that advanced into cancer, showing a huge diversity in types of colorectal cancer and genetic involvement.

In 1882 W. Harrison Cripps associated in his work that multiple intestinal polyposis had hereditary nature and also potentially malignant nature. Subsequently in 1913 Aldred S. Warthin reported on 1600 cases of carcinoma treated at University of Michigan for 19 years, collecting detailed family histories of approximately 500 patients and mapping a predisposition to gastrointestinal and endometrial carcinogenesis of three generations. In 1950, Eldon J. Gardner at University of Utah conducted a long genetic study in patient families with multiple polyps and established a link between this event and a predisposition to carcinomatosis only in 1986 Herrera et al. described a case of a patient with polyposis and multiple carcinomatosis, with an amputation in a long arm of chromosome 5, suggesting a location of tumor suppressor gene. Subsequent studies in families with polyps have identified the 5q21 region as adenomatous polyposis coli or APC gene. Since then, we have identified numerous genetic defects and genetic expressions showing a diversity of mutations with distinct pathways of progression [2].

There have been significant advances in the last years and more than understanding the risk factors for CCR, recent progress in the field of molecular biology, has allowed us to identify the oncogenesis basis to the development of the disease. Then apply these knowledge in the research of new drugs that lead to better outcomes even in the advanced disease.

2. Molecular basis of carcinogenesis in colorectal cancer

In medical practice, patients with cancer present with great frequency, clinical evolution in a differentiated way in response to the treatment performed. As a result, there is a high margin of uncertainty as to the effectuation of the treatment performed, not infrequently counting initially favorable prognostic evaluations [3].

Cancer results from a long process of at least three phases: initiation, promotion and progression, which reflect accumulated genetic alterations, responsible for the transformation of normal cells into neoplastic cells. The mechanisms of transformation of a normal cell into neoplastic involve a number of genetic and molecular events that affect proliferation and differentiation. In the pathogenesis of neoplastic processes, two groups of genes are involved: proto-oncogenes, which stimulate cell growth and impede differentiation, and tumor suppressor genes, which promote differentiation and limit cell proliferation. The imbalance in the regulation of this system, through the activation of proto-oncogenes or loss of the function of tumor suppressor genes, can lead to the uncontrolled proliferation of cells and to the accumulation of successive genetic abnormalities characteristic of neoplastic cells [4–7].

The development of cancer (oncogenesis) results from mutations in one or more genes, responsible for the regulation of cell growth and programmed cell death called apoptosis (**Figure 1**) [8]. When cancer occurs as part of a hereditary cancer syndrome, the initial mutation causing the cancer is inherited through germ lineage. However, most cancers are sporadic because mutations occur in a single somatic cell, which then divides and proceeds to develop cancer [9].

Considering a frequency of 10-10 replication errors per DNA basis, cell division, and about 1015 cell divisions over the life span of an adult, only replication errors would result in thousands of mutations in the DNA of the genome [8].

Once initiated, a cancer progresses through additional accumulation of genetic damage through mutations in maintenance genes, which encode the DNA repairing cellular machinery. Changes in these genes produce mutations in increasing numbers, leading to failures in controlling cell proliferation and repairing DNA damage. In this way, the original clone of neoplastic cells functions as a reservoir of genetically unstable cells, known as cancer stem cells. These give rise to multiple underlining of varying degrees of malignancy, each carrying a set of mutations. In this context, cancer is a multifactorial disease with an important genetic component, and mutations are central to its etiology and progression [8] (**Figure 2**).

The classical CCR carcinogenesis model is based on the adenoma-carcinoma sequence in which tumor onset occurs from a sequential and progressive process. This involves the activation of oncogenesis (K-ras) and the inactivation of tumor suppressor genes (APC, DCC, p53) [10, 11]. This model of carcinogenesis, where there is chromosomal instability, is usually found in the distal segments of the colon and rectum [11]. The adenoma-carcinoma sequence was described for the first time by Hill et al. (**Figure 3**) [12].

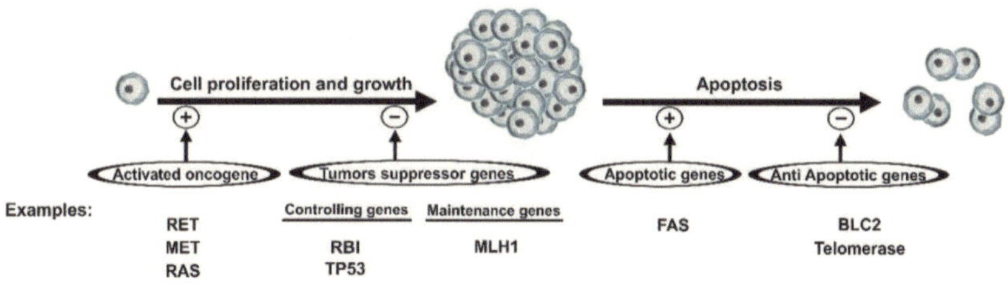

Figure 1.
Mechanism of oncogenesis. General scheme for mechanism of oncogenesis by proto-oncogene activation, loss of tumor suppressor gene expression, activation of anti-apoptotic genes or loss of pro-apoptotic gene expression. The effect of the genes that induce a process is shown as +, while the effect of the genes that suppress a process is shown as −. Modified from Thompson and Thompson [8].

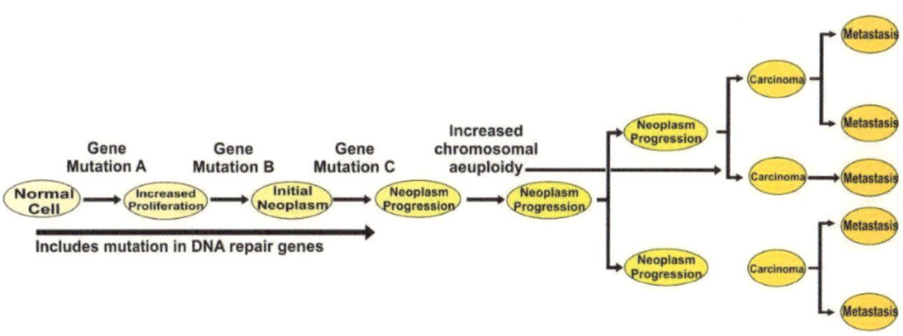

Figure 2.
Stages in the evolution of cancer. Increasing degrees of abnormalities are associated with sequential loss of tumor suppressor genes from various chromosomes and activation of proto-oncogenes, with or without a defect, concomitant in DNA repair. Modified from Thompson and Thompson [8].

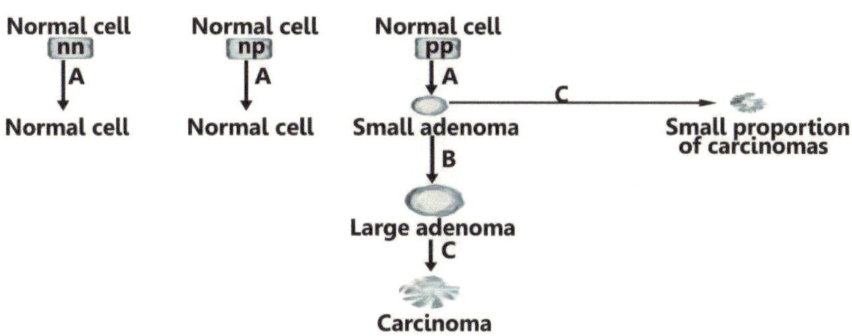

Figure 3.
The adenoma-carcinoma sequence. Postulated mechanism for progression from normal tissue to adenoma to carcinoma. n: normal gene; p: adenoma gene (recessive), so that cell pp: is adenoma-prone. A: environmental agent causing adenomas only in adenoma-prone cell. B: environmental agent causing adenomas to grow. C: agent causing adenomas to develop into carcinomas. Modified from Hill et al. [12].

In the colorectal carcinogenesis, there are a complex interaction between environmental and lifestyle factors and multiple molecular pathways contributes to its occurrence. Three different molecular mechanisms are implicated in colorectal carcinogenesis: chromosomal instability (CIN), genetic instability (GIN) and the serrated pathway. However, although they differ at the beginning of the chain of events, their signaling pathway, implicated in the transformation of the normal epithelial colorectal cell to the neoplastic one, appear to be similar and converge to the clinical and pathological manifestation of the disease. These genetic mechanisms can be acquired after birth and the occurrence of cancer is called sporadic or they can be inherited from the genitors and in this case is called hereditary. In the recent past, only clinical and pathological manifestations were considered when proposing the optimal treatment. However, after the understanding of the patterns implicated in the carcinogenesis, the tumors could be classificated according to molecular standards and individual treatment schemes were developed [13].

2.1 Chromosomal instability

The most frequent model of phenotype group in colorectal cancer are allelic losses in the short arm of chromosome 17 and 8 and in the long arm of chromosomes 5, 18 and 22, being approximately 80% of the sporadic form and are related to mutations in tumor suppressor genes of TP53 genes, APC, SMAD2, and SMAD4.

The first major accepted model for cancer development in colon was described by Fearon and Vogelstein in 1990. The majority of the sporadic CCR tumors originates from premalignant precursor lesions known as polyps, which over time progress to clinically relevant tumors. In this model, the sequence of events leading from the adenoma (polyps) to carcinoma was based on mutation on APC and TP53 genes [13, 14].

The proto-oncogene K-ras (Kirsten-ras) tumor suppressor genes, APC protein (adenomatous polyposis coli), DCC protein (deleted in colorectal cancer) and TP53; and DNA repair or mismatch repair genes (MSH2, MLH1, PMS1, PMS2 and MSH6) are fundamental in development of CCR. Repetitive nucleotide sequences form approximately 25–40% of the DNA molecule being observed several times across the genome as dispersed replicates and tandem or satellite replicates [15]. These replicates can be classified according to the extension of the repetitive sequence in: satellite, minisatellite and microsatellite, depending on the number of nucleotides [16].

Most of the cases of CCR originate from polyps, but it was evidenced that about 45% of the tumors located in the proximal colon originated from epithelium without preexisting polyps, being considered new cancer [17]. In this model of carcinogenesis, which affects 10–15% of cases of sporadic CCR, instead of chromosomal instability there would be genomic instability due to mutations of DNA repair proteins, a phenomenon known as microsatellite instability (IMS) [18]. This pathway of colorectal carcinogenesis due to chromosomal instability is more frequently observed in tumors in the proximal colon, presenting characteristic histological features, being diploid, exophytic growth, worse histological grade, greater tendency to mucus production and lower mutation index in the TP53 gene, and paradoxically, they are associated with a better prognosis [18, 19].

2.2 Microsatellite instability

DNA is a molecule that often undergoes changes through loss of segments, mutations that occur during the process of cell division. To correct these changes, it has proteins with the function of performing the repairs necessary to maintain its integrity. These proteins are produced from some genes known as repair (mismatch repair genes—MMR) and this function is carried out continuously, preserving the cellular tissues [20–22]. The hMLH1 gene is located on chromosome 3p21-23 [23, 24], hMSH2 on chromosome 2p21 [25–27] and hMSH6 is on 2p16 [28].

In hereditary CCR there are two genetic pathways of carcinogenesis: a chromosomal instability pathway, which occurs in PAF (familial adenomatous polyposis), where the patient inherits a mutation of the APC (adenomatous colonic polyposis) tumor suppressor gene, and DNA hypermutability pathway, which occurs in HNPCC (inherited non-polyposis colorectal cancer) in which the inherited genetic change is the inactivation of one of the alleles of genes involved in DNA repair (hMSH2 and hMLH1 genes). However, other genes are involved in colorectal carcinogenesis, such as K-ras gene, DCC gene, Tp53 gene, etc. [29].

DNA is a molecule that often undergoes changes through loss of segments, mutations that occur during the process of cell division. To correct these changes, it has proteins with the function of performing the repairs necessary to maintain its integrity. These proteins are produced from some genes known as repair (mismatch repair genes—MMR) and this function is carried out continuously, preserving the cellular tissues [20–22]. The hMLH1 gene is located on chromosome 3p21-23 [23, 24], hMSH2 on chromosome 2p21 [25–27] and hMSH6 is on 2p16 [28].

MMRs have the function of recognizing the occurrence of the mutation and blocking cell division in order to prevent the emergence of a defective cell line, which is done by inducing cell death (apoptosis) or performing DNA repair. For the latter, these proteins remove a segment of DNA containing the change and insert a new segment containing the right sequence, based on the "template" of the complementary DNA [30].

The failure of these proteins to function will cause a great instability in the genome, that is, defects in the sequence of base pairs occurring at random in DNA replication cannot be adequately repaired, generating an accumulation of genetic abnormalities that favor the emergence of cancer [30].

A genetic instability that appears in 12–15% of CCR cases, named MSI (microsatellite instability) as a result of a mismatch repair (MMR), what leading to the accumulation of mutations in genes controlling cell cycle and apoptosis (TGFBRII, BAX or CASPASE5) [31].

Cells with changes in MMRs are not able to correctly repair errors during DNA replication. Because of their repetitive structure, microsatellite regions in DNA are particularly prone to these repair errors [32, 33]. The DNA of cells of certain tumors presents differences in the number of repetitive units in one or more microsatellites, when compared to the same microsatellites in the DNA of normal cells, a fact called microsatellite instability (MSI). as positive for replication errors, that is, RER (+) [34].

More than 90% of HNPCC patients present RER (+), while about 15% of sporadic CCRs present this genetic trait [30].

Repair proteins in their normal state form heterodimers [35–38]. MSH2 dimerizes with MSH6 forming the MutSα [38] functional complex, and MLH1 dimerizes with PMS2 to form MutLα [37, 39]. It has been shown that MSH2 and MLH1 proteins are obligatory parts of their respective heterodimers [40–42]. Their abnormalities may result in a proteolytic degradation of their dimers and consequently loss of both mandatory and secondarily associated proteins, the exception includes only MLH1 mutations, when the mutations result in the antigenically activation of the mutated MLH1 protein, which may be the loss of PMS2 only. The reverse, however, is not true, when mutation occurs in the genes of secondary proteins, for example, in MSH6 and PMS2, loss of MSH2 and MLH1 proteins that may not occur, inasmuch as other proteins compensate the function of the secondary proteins, such as MSH3, MLH3 and PMS1. In effect, mutations of MLH1 or MSH2 routinely cause loss of MLH1/PMS2 or MSH2/MHS6, respectively, while mutations of PMS2 or MSH6 cause isolated loss of PMS2 or MSH2 only [43].

Figure 4 shows the model of DNA repair proteins in patients with colorectal cancer [44].

Studies performed in CCR demonstrated a positivity index for greater microsatellite instability in young patients or located in proximal segments of the colon. A study restricted to rectum tumors, the incidence of repair errors was only in 2% of cases, confirming the relationship between microsatellite instability and tumors located in the right or transverse colon [45]. The CCR associated with repair errors tend to present the same location and biological behavior independent of their sporadic or hereditary nature (HNPCC) [45].

2.3 Serrated pathway

The serrated pathway was first described by Longacre and Fenoglio-Preiser in 1990 and differs from the classical adenoma-carcinoma sequence one because in this way there is the participation of other genetic alterations other than chromosomal instability and KRAS mutations like BRAF mutations and gene promoter hypermethylation. But in the serrated pathway, microsatellite instability can also be detected.

The serrated polyps are characterized by glandular serration in which the colonic epithelial crypts show luminal "saw-toothed" pattern. The nomenclature is not well established but the World Health Organization in 2010 classified them into three main groups: hyperplastic polyps, sessile serrated adenomas/polyps and traditional serrated adenomas [46].

Genetically, carcinoma arising from serrated polyps are MSI-H and shows epithelial serrations, clear, eosinophilic and abundant cytoplasm, vesicular nuclei, absence of necrosis, mucin production and presence of cell balls and rods. The finding of serrated lesion in the peripheral of an invasive carcinoma also leads to the diagnostic of this pathway.

Serrated adenocarcinoma is found in about 10% of sporadic colorectal cancers and is originated in the serrated polyp-carcinoma pathway. In this way, hyperplastic polyps now are recognized as neoplastic lesions because they may predispose

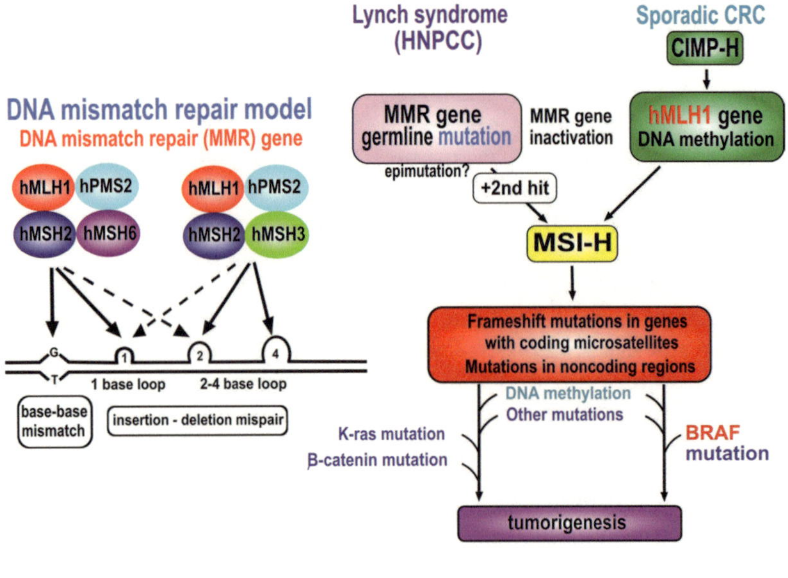

Figure 4.
Model of DNA repair proteins and molecular pathways for CCR with microsatellite instability. Modified from Kohzoh and Yamamoto [44].

to cancer in a sequence in which they progress to serrated adenomas and then to colorectal cancer in at about 7 years. It is not clear why only a few groups of hyperplastic polyps, mainly the ones located in the right colon, will progress to carcinoma and the answer is probably dependent on the genetic findings not elucidated until now. A great number of studies have shown that the right colon is not the same organ as the left colon and the right-sided cancer tends to be more aggressive and this difference is caused by the difference of genetic standard between the sides.

The clinical management of hyperplastic polyps and serrated polyps is essential for avoiding the carcinoma transformation. The most important procedure for prophylaxis is the complete removal of these polyps in colonoscopy and the subsequent surveillance but it is not well established how to follow up. Just for comparison, in the classical adenomatous polyps, the size, number and histological variants (if tubular, villous or tubulovillous) are taken in account to determine the interval of surveillance and this knowledge is more than a decade old. For serrated polyps, as the understanding of this pattern of via is recent, the follow up is not clear hence studies have not shown yet which features are important to determine the risk of progression of these lesions. Moreover, the majority of serrated polyps will not progress to carcinoma and studies answering why are not yet available. A few studies have demonstrated that sessile serrated lesions larger than 10 mm are at high risk for carcinoma progress. But despite the lack of information and in order to prevent cancer arising via serrated pathway, the complete removal of serrated polyps is the goal in these cases.

If there are significant differences regarding the genetic markers and pathological findings in serrated pathway, it is expected to have differences in the presentation of the disease and response to therapy. And some evidences have showed these: carcinomas arising from serrated pathway tends to have lesser 5-year survival but again the causes of this comportment are not available, and the answer may be found as the genetic alterations becomes evident [47].

For now, it is clear that serrated pathway is a well-established pattern that explains the behavior of some hyperplastic and serrated polyps that could not have been explained in the classical adenoma-carcinoma sequence using CIN and MSI models. Even with lacks in knowledge for profound understanding, the pathological and molecular characterization of these polyps are constantly progressing and studies in the next few years will probably show the best way to manage these cases in clinical practice [47].

3. Conclusion

There have been significant advances about tumor molecular biology, will allow us to apply this knowledge in more specific diagnostic techniques, a proper diagnosis, with the possibility of detecting earlier pre-malignant lesions and diagnoses. This applied research knowledge would allow the development of more efficient therapies for cancer, moreover, it can act in prevention.

The application of molecular biology knowledge in the diagnosis and treatment of colorectal cancer generates a great impact on the accuracy of diagnosis and optimization of cancer therapy in order to individualize the treatment, thereby trying to reduce the uncertainty about the effectiveness of the treatment that will be accomplished.

Author details

Lenuce Ribeiro Aziz Ydy[1*], Willian Ricardo Camarço-Silva[1]
and Wilson Vilela Medeiros-Filho[2]

1 Federal University of Mato Grosso, Cuiabá, State of Mato Grosso, Brazil

2 Hospital Municipal Milton Pessoa Morbeck, Barra Do Garças, Mato Grosso, Brazil

*Address all correspondence to: lenuceydy@gmail.com

References

[1] American Institute for Cancer Research [homepage on internet]. Colorectal Cancer Statistics. Available from: https://www.wcrf.org/dietandcancer/cancer-trends/colorectal-cancer-statistics [Accessed: 05 February 2019]

[2] Hankey W, Groden J. The genetics of colorectal cancer. In: Haigis KM, editor. Molecular Pathogenesis of Colorectal Cancer. New York: Springer; 2013. pp. 1-24

[3] Pinho MSL. Estadiamento molecular do cancer colorretal: o future se aproxima. Revista Brasileira de Coloproctologia. 2005;**25**(3):271-284

[4] Tsongalis GJ, Coleman WB. Molecular oncology: Diagnostic and prognostic assessment of human cancers in the clinical laboratory. Cancer Investigation. 1998;**16**(7):485-502

[5] Bain B. Diagnóstico Em Leucemias. 2ª ed. Rio de Janeiro: Revinter; 2003

[6] Felsher DW. Reversibility of oncogene-induced cancer. Current Opinion in Genetics & Development. 2004;**14**(1):37-42

[7] Robbins S. Patologia Estrutural e Funcional. Rio de Janeiro: Guanabara Koogan; 2000

[8] Thompsoson JS, Thompson MW. Genética Médica. Rio de Janeiro: Guanabara; 2007

[9] Ydy LRA, Damazo AS, Dicke E, Ydy RRA. Biologia molecular em oncologia. In: Figueiredo EMA, Correia MM, Oliveira AF, editors. Tratado de Oncologia. 1ª ed. Rio de Janeiro: Revinter; 2013. pp. 43-52

[10] Volgelstein B, Fearon ER, Hamilton SR, Kern SE, Preisinger AC, Leppert M, et al. Genetic alterations during colorectal tumor development. The New England Journal of Medicine. 1988;**319**(9):525-532

[11] Fearon ER, Volgelstein B. A genetic model for colorectal tumorigenesis. Cell. 1990;**61**(5):759-767

[12] Hill MJ, Morson BC, Bussey HJ. A etiology of adenoma-carcinoma sequence in large-bowel. Lancet. 1978;**1**:245-247

[13] Tariq K, Ghias K. Colorectal cancer carcinogenesis: A review of mechanisms. Cancer Biology & Medicine. 2016;**13**(1):120-135. DOI: 10.28092/j.issn.2095-3941.2015.0103

[14] Laurent-Puig P, Agostini J, Maley K. Oncogenèse colorectale. Bulletin du Cancer. 2010;**97**(11):1311-1321. DOI: 10.1684/bdc.2010.1216

[15] Cutait R, Cotti G, Garicochea B, Muraro C, Carvalho F, Leite K, et al. Instabilidade de microssatélites em portadores de câncer colo-retal. Revista Brasileira de Coloproctologia. 2002;**4**:225-232

[16] Abe Y, Masuda H, Okubo R. Microsatellite instability of each tumor in sporadic synchronous multiple colorectal cancers. Oncology Reports. 2001;**8**(2):299-304

[17] Bedenne L, Faivre J, Boutron MC, Piard F, Cauvin JM, Hillon P. Adenoma-carcinoma sequence or "de novo" carcinogenesis? A study of adenomatous remnants in a population-based series of large bowel cancers. Cancer. 1992;**69**(4):883-888

[18] Kim H, Jen J, Volgelstein B, Hamilton SR. Clinical and pathological characteristics of sporadic colorectal carcinomas with DNA replication errors in microsatellite sequences. The American Journal of Pathology. 1994;**145**(1):148-156

[19] Martinez CAR, Priolli DG, Cardinalli IA, Pereira JA, Portes AV, Margarido NF. Influência da localização do tumor na expressão tecidual da proteína p53 em doentes com câncer colorretal Estudo de 100 casos. Revista do Colégio Brasileiro de Cirurgiões. 2008;**35**(4):235-243

[20] Gervaz P, Cerottini JP, Bouzourene H, Hahnloser D, Doan CL, Benhattar J, et al. Comparison of microsatellite instability and chromosomal instability in predicting survival of patients with T3N0 colorectal cancer. Surgery. 2002;**131**(2):190-197

[21] Grizzle WE, Shibata D, Manne U, Myers RB, Frost AR. Molecular, and histopathologic changes in the development of colorectal neoplasia. In: Srivastava S, Henson DE, Gazdar A, editors. Molecular Pathology of Early Cancer. Chapter 10. Amsterdam, Netherlands: IOS Press; 1999. pp. 135-170

[22] Wang JYJ, Edelmann W. Mismatch repair proteins as sensors of alkylation DNA damage. Cancer Cell. 2006;**9**:417-418

[23] Jeon CH, Lee HI, Shin IH, Park JW. Genetic alterations of APC, K-ras, p53, MSI, and MAGE in Korean colorectal cancer patients. International Journal of Colorectal Disease. 2008;**23**(1):29-35

[24] Kashyap VK, Sitalaximi T, Chattopadhyay P, Trivedi R. Dna profiling tecnologies in forensis analysis. International Journal of Human Genetics. 2004;**4**(1):11-30

[25] Nyström-Lahti M, Sistonen P, Mecklin JP, Pylkkänen L, Aaltonen LA, Järvinen H, et al. Close linkage to chromosome 3p and conservation of ancestral founding haplotype in hereditary nonpolyposis colorectal cancer families. Proceedings of the National Academy of Sciences of the United States of America. 1994;**91**(13):6054-6058

[26] Pinho MSL. Biologia molecular no câncer colorretal: um corte atual na literatura. Revista Brasileira de Coloproctologia. 2002;**22**(4):284-288

[27] Lewin B. Gene VII. Artemed: Porto Alegre; 2001

[28] Terui H, Tachikawa T, Kakuta M, Nishimura Y, Yatsuoka T, Yamaguchi K, et al. Molecular and clinical characteristics of MSH5 germline variants detects in colorectal cancer patients. Oncology Reports. 2013;**30**(6):2909-2916

[29] Vogelstein B, Fearon ER, Kern SE, Hamilton SR, Preisinger AC, Nakamura Y, et al. Allelotype of colorectal carcinomas. Science. 1989;**244**:207-211

[30] Pinho MSL, Rossi BM. As proteínas envolvidas na carcinogênes colorretal (IV). Revista Brasileira de Coloproctologia. 1998;**18**(4):278-282

[31] Yamane L, Scapulatempo-Neto C, Reis RM, Guimarães DP. Serrated pathway in colorectal carcinogenesis. World Journal of Gastroenterology. 14 March 2014;**20**(10):2634-2640. DOI: 10.3748/wjg.v20.i10.2634

[32] Zhou XP, Hoang JM, Li YJ, et al. Determination of the replication error phenotype in human tumors without the requirement for matching normal DNA by analysis of mononucleotide repeat microsatellites. Genes, Chromosomes & Cancer. 1998;**21**:101-107

[33] Hoang JM, Cottu PH, Thuille B, Salmon RJ, Thomas G, Hamelin R. Bat-26, an indicator of the replication error phenotype in colorectal cancers and cell lines. Cancer Research. 1997;**57**:300-303

[34] Oliveira VC, Leite SMO, Gomes KB, Ferreira ACS, Pardini VC. A importância do estudo de instabilidade

de microssatélite na avalição do câncer colorretal hereditário não polipose (HNPCC). NeusLab. 2005;**73**:115-118

[35] Jacur T, Boland CR. Structure and function of the components of the human DNA mismatch repair system. International Journal of Cancer. 2006;**119**:2030-2035

[36] Fishel R. The selection for mismatch repair defects in hereditary nonpolyposis colorectal câncer: Revising the mutator hypothesis. Cancer Research. 2001;**61**:7369-7374

[37] Kadyrov FA, Dzantiev L, Constantin N, Modrich P. Endonucleolytic function of MutLalpha in human mismatch repair. Cell. 2006;**126**:297-308

[38] Acharya S, Wilson T, Gradia S, Kane MF, Guerrette S, Marsischky GT, et al. hMSH2 and hMSH6 forms specific mispair-binding complexes with hMSH3 and hMSH6. Proceedings of the National Academy of Sciences of the United States of America. 1996;**93**:13629-13634

[39] Harfe BD, Minesinger BK, Jinks-Robertson S. Discrete in vivo roles for the MutL homologs Mlh2p and Mlh3p in removal of frameshift intermediates in budding yeast. Current Biology. 2000;**10**:145-148

[40] de Jong AE, van Puijenbroek M, Hendriks Y, Tops C, Wijnen J, Ausems MG, et al. Microsatellite instability, immunohistochemistry, and additional PMS2 staining in suspected hereditary nonpolyposis colorectal cancer. Clinical Cancer Research. 2004;**10**:972-980

[41] Umar A, Koi M, Risinger JI, Glaab WE, Tindall KR, Kolodner RD, et al. Correction of hypermutability, N-methyl-N'-nitro-N-nitrosoguanidine resistance, and defective DNA mismatch repair by introducing chromosome 2 into human tumor cells with mutations in MSH2 and MSH6. Cancer Research. 1997;**57**:3949-3955

[42] Watanabe Y, Haugen-Strano A, Umar Yamada K, Hemmi H, Kikuchi Y, Takano S, et al. Complementation of an hMSH2 defect in human colorectal carcinoma cells by human chromosome 2 transfer. Molecular Carcinogenesis. 2000;**29**:37-49

[43] Shia J. Immunohistochemistry versus microsatellite instability testing for screening colorectal cancer patients at risk for hereditary nonpolyposis colorectal cancer syndrome. Part I. Utility of immunohistochemistry. The Journal of Molecular Diagnostics. 2008;**10**(4):293-300

[44] Kohzoh I, Yamamoto H. Carcinogenesis and microsatellite instability: The interrelationship between genetics and epigenetics. Carcinogenesis. 2008;**29**(4):673-680

[45] Pinho MSL. Câncer colorretal com instabilidade de microssatélites: Uma doença diferente. Revista Brasileira de Coloproctologia. 2002;**22**(2):139-144

[46] Szylberg L, Janiczek M, Popiel A, Marszałek A. Serrated polyps and their alternative pathway to the colorectal cancer: A systematic review. Gastroenterology Research and Practice.2015;**2015**:573814, 1-7. DOI: 10.1155/2015/573814

[47] Nojadeh JN, Sharif SB, Sakhinia E. Microsatellite instability in colorectal cancer. EXCLI Journal. 2018;**17**:159-168. ISSN: 1611-2156. DOI: 10.17179/excli2017-948

Section 4

Multidisciplinary Approach for Treating Colorectal Cancer

Chapter 4

Targeted Photodynamic Therapy as Potential Treatment Modality for the Eradication of Colon Cancer

Cherie Ann Kruger and Heidi Abrahamse

Abstract

Photodynamic therapy (PDT) can be used to treat colorectal cancer (CRC). When a photosensitizer (PS) drug is administered to a patient, it can either passively or actively accumulate within a tumor site and once exposed to a specific wavelength of light, it is excited to produce reactive oxygen species (ROS), resulting in tumor destruction. However, the efficacy of ROS generation for tumor damage is highly dependent on the uptake of the PS in tumor cells. Thus, PS targeted uptake and delivery in CRC tumor cells is a crucial factor in PDT cancer drug absorption studies. Generally, within non-targeted drug delivery mechanisms, only minor amounts of PS passively accumulate in tumor sites and the remainder distributes into healthy tissues, causing unwanted side effects. To improve the efficacy of PDT research is currently focused on the development of specific receptor based photosynthetic nanocarrier platform drugs, which promote the active uptake and absorption of PS drugs in CRC tumor sites only, avoiding unwanted side effects, as well as treatment enhancement. This chapter will focus on current actively targeted PS nanoparticle drug delivery systems, which have been investigated for the PDT treatment of CRC cancer.

Keywords: colorectal cancer, photodynamic therapy, photosensitizer, nanoparticles, targeted drug delivery

1. Introduction: colorectal cancer (CRC)

There are over a million new cases of colorectal cancer (CRC) being diagnosed worldwide each year [1]. CRC is known to be the third most commonly diagnosed cancer malignancy worldwide and is the fourth most frequent cause of cancer related cell deaths, with around 0.6 million deaths annually [2].

CRC is an uncontrolled growth that originates within polyps that are found in the inner lining of either the colon or rectum [3]. The intestinal wall of the colon and rectum is made up of many layers [3]. CRC polyp growth formation begins within the innermost mucosal layers of either the colon or rectum and these polyps can grow outward through some or all of these intestinal layers [1]. When CRC primary polyp cells growth spreads from the inner to the outer intestinal walls, they can grow into blood or lymph vessels and so spread to other parts of the body forming secondary cancer metastasizes [1]. Adenocarcinomas polyps originate within intestinal cells that produce mucus to lubricate the inside of either the colon or rectum and this is the most common form of CRC, with approximately 96% of cases, being diagnosed annually [3]. Other less common types of CRC tumors that can originate in colorectal tissues or cells include: lymphomas, sarcomas, gastrointestinal carcinoid or stromal tumors [3].

The risk of developing of CRC is often attributed to either a variety of environmental factors or genetic predispositions. Approximately 25% of diagnosed CRC cases can be attributed to inherited syndromes, while the remaining 75% cases are due to external environmental contributing factors [4, 5]. The most common CRC inherited syndromes include familial adenomatous polyposis (FAP) and hereditary nonpolyposis colorectal cancers (HNPCC) [4]. While common triggering environmental factors include: diets which are low in fiber and high in fat and red meat, low physical activity, obesity, heavy alcohol consumption, cigarette smoking and deskbound seated occupations [5].

Even though numerous advances have been made in relation to early diagnosis and treatment of CRC, tumor reoccurrence and metastatic spread are two critical factors which affect the survival rate of patients [6]. Dependent on the stage at which they have been diagnosed, approximately 25% of patients with CRC at time of diagnosis have metastases (due to late detection) and 50% of patients diagnosed with CRC will develop metastases, either at presentation or during follow-up [7, 8].

2. Resistance of CRC to conventional treatments

The most common conventional treatments for CRC include surgical resection, chemotherapy or radiation therapy [9]. These treatments are either used in combination or alone depending on the stage at which the disease has been detected and diagnosed [9].

In early stages (0 to I) of CRC diagnosis, the most common treatment practice is surgical resection of the CRC polyps, without any further need for treatment [10]. In stages II to III of CRC detection, surgical resection with lymph node dissection to examine for presence of cancer cell spread, is standard practice [11]. Patients with stage IV CRC disease often require chemotherapy and/or radiation therapy combined with surgery to treat the disease [12].

Typical standard CRC chemotherapy treatment regimens include; FOLFOX: leucovorin, 5-fluorouracil (5-FU), and oxaliplatin (Eloxatin), FOLFIRI: leucovorin, 5-FU, and irinotecan (Camptosar), CAPEOX or CAPOX: capecitabine (Xeloda) and oxaliplatin, FOLFOXIRI: leucovorin, 5-FU, oxaliplatin, and irinotecan, one of the previous combinations, plus either a drug that targets VEGF, (bevacizumab [Avastin], ziv-aflibercept [Zaltrap], or ramucirumab [Cyramza]), or a drug that targets EGFR (cetuximab [Erbitux] or panitumumab [Vectibix]) or 5-FU and leucovorin, with or without a targeted drug, Capecitabine, with or without a targeted drug, Irinotecan, with or without a targeted drug, Cetuximab alone, Panitumumab alone, Regorafenib (Stivarga) alone, Trifluridine and tipiracil (Lonsurf) [13].

Thus, 5-FU-based chemotherapy remains the mainstay of therapy for patients with CRC, however in recent year's chemotherapy drugs such as oxaliplatin, irinotecan and capecitabine have been developed and generally conventional chemotherapy treatment for advanced CRC combines 5-FU and leucovorin with oxaliplatin or irinotecan [14]. The greatest strides over recent years in chemotherapy treatments have been combining these drugs with monoclonal antibodies such as Bevacizumab and Cetuximab in order to target vascular endothelial growth factor (VEGF) or epidermal growth factor receptor (EGFR) which are respectively overexpressed in CRC cells [14, 15]. Angiogenesis, plays an important role in CRC tumor development and metastasis, is partly mediated by vascular endothelial growth factor (VEGF), thus by combining chemotherapeutic drugs with Bevacizumab monoclonal antibodies, VEGF overexpressed receptors can be targeted to enhance drug uptake and so improve treatment [14, 15]. Likewise, since EGFR plays and important role in tumorigenesis, it is often found to be overexpressed in a high percentage of patients with late-stage colorectal cancer and by combining chemotherapeutic drugs with Cetuximab monoclonal antibodies, chemotherapeutic drug targeting and uptake can be promoted [14, 15]. Moreover, by utilizing chemotherapy monoclonal antibody treatments for CRC, resistance to EGFR inhibitors may be partially mediated, by activating VEGF-dependent signaling, and so drug delivery strategies that combine anti-EGFR and anti-VEGF agents appear promising [15].

Overall, the choice of these various chemotherapy treatment regimens for CRC depends on various factors such as previous treatments received, if the regime is no longer working and the patients overall health [13]. For some patients with certain genetic marker changes in their CRC cells another treatment option after chemotherapy to be considered is immunotherapy with pembrolizumab [13].

Nevertheless, despite the improved CRC response rates with these various advanced strategies, the overall survival rate for metastatic CRC remains only slightly over 12% [18]. One of the major causes for this poor survival rate is due to the fact that nearly half of all metastatic CRC patients are resistant to 5-FU-based chemotherapies, which demises their overall treatment and recovery [14]. The reason for the development of chemotherapeutic drug resistance in CRC cells is that they have the ability to enhance DNA repair mechanisms, deregulate signaling pathways, as well as increase drug metabolism [16]. Generally, 90% CRC patients report drug resistance to chemotherapies, resulting in poor treatment due to oncogene mutations, which deregulate signaling pathways [16]. This deregulation of signaling pathways, results in increased aerobic glycolysis, fatty acid synthesis, and glutamine metabolism causing a decrease in chemotherapeutic drug induced apoptosis [17]. Moreover, drug efflux transporter proteins are often found to be overexpressed in drug-resistant CRC cells, which decrease the successful uptake of chemotherapeutic drugs in cancer cells [6, 18]. Thus, if metastases has occurred, chemotherapy will probably not be curative and so only help in improving prognosis via tumor shrinkage [19]. Thus continuous research is required into CRC in order to unravel these multiple drug resistance mechanisms and so develop improved treatment regimens with better outcomes [18, 19].

Radiation therapy is usually utilized pre-CRC surgical resection in stages II to IV, depending on the degree of metastasis, to shrink un-respectable tumors or to try and help control the cancer that has spread to other parts of the body [11, 20]. However, radiation therapy has numerous unwanted side effects in patients receiving such treatments, which include: nausea, stool leakage, fatigue, sexual problems, skin irritation, rectal irritation and diarrhea [21]. Moreover, some CRC patients have noted resistance to radiation therapy, whereby in response to radiation DNA damage, Ataxia Telangiectasia Mutated (ATM) genes and anti-apoptotic factors phosphatases of regenerating liver-3 (PRL-3) become activated in cancer cells and so begin to regulate cancer cell pro-survival and resistance [22]. Additionally, these genes have been noted to be overexpressed in CRC patients whom have previously received radiation therapy and their cancer has reoccurred, shortening their survival [23].

Moreover, in addition to resistance to conventional treatments, the metastasis spread of CRC is of major concern. Primary CRC tumors are highly prone to TGF-β, PIK3CA, and TP53 gene mutations and since these genes are responsible for clonal expansion and invasiveness, the metastatic cellular potential of CRC to spread is high [24]. Lastly, another important factor in CRCs resistance to conventional therapies and metastasis, is the presence of cancer stem cells, since these cells have the ability to go by undetected (due to their slow growth) and so enhances CRC treatment resistance, as well as allows this type of cancer to initiate new tumor growth and so metastasize [6].

Thus, currently conventional treatments are not very successful at curing CRC and patients are at high risk of developing secondary cancers, due to the ease at which this cancer can migrate through the blood and lymphatic systems to other parts of the body, such as the liver, lungs and digestive system [8, 25]. Thus, there is dire need to investigate other alternative therapies for the treatment of CRC.

3. Photodynamic therapy an unconventional treatment for CRC

Photodynamic therapy (PDT) is a promising unconventional treatment method for CRC (**Figure 1**) [8].

PDT treatment is a coordinated process, which begins with the intravenous administration of a photosensitizer (PS) drug [8]. Once the PS drug enters the blood stream it is then either passively or actively absorbed in tumor site, depending on the PS drug delivery mechanism that is involved [26]. Within standard conventional PS drug delivery mechanisms the advantage is that the PS drug tend to preferentially localize in diseased tissue via the enhanced permeability retention (EPR) effect and so is passively absorbed, promoting PDT induced tumor destruction with only slight healthy tissue damage [26]. However, current research studies are focused on improving PS passive drug uptake via chemical or functional modifications in order to promote a more specific and actively targeted PS delivery in cancer cells only, so that photosensitivity, localized healthy tissue destruction and other additional unwanted side effects can possibly be eliminated [26]. Since, PS drugs are light absorbing molecules their activation is achieved when they are

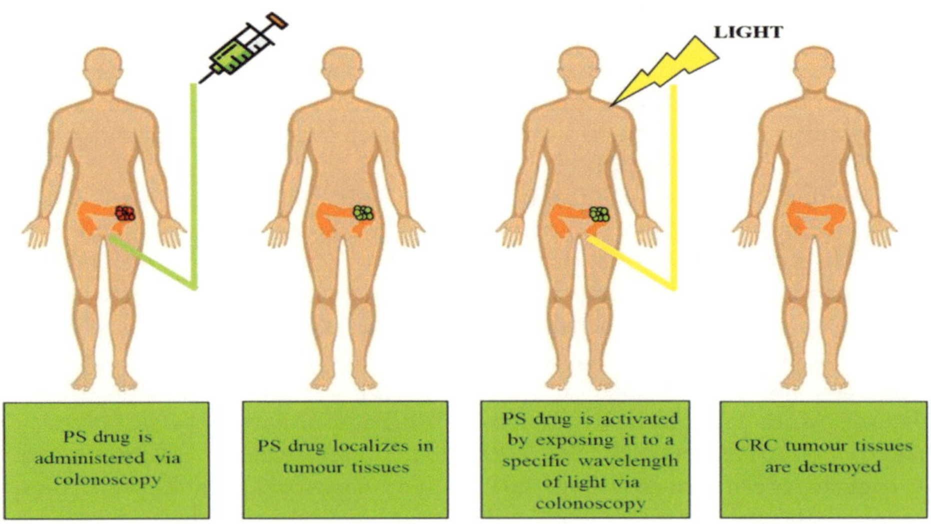

Figure 1.
PDT treatment of CRC. PS drugs are administered to a patients CRC tumor site via a colonoscopy endoscope, whereby they localize in targeted tumor cells. Laser light irradiation is then also administered to the target tumor site via a colonoscopy endoscope, whereby it penetrates the large intestines tissues/tumor and activates the PS. The PS then undergoes a photoreaction to produce ROS and/or singlet oxygen, which in turn induces cytotoxic cell death in CRC tumor tissues.

exposed to laser irradiation light at a specific wavelength [26]. Thus when a tumor (which contains the localized PS drug) is exposed to laser irradiation light, the PS absorbs the photons and becomes excited [2]. This excitation promotes the PS from a ground state to a higher level of energy known as a singlet state [27]. This singlet state is very short lived and PSs return to their ground state rapidly after losing their energy to fluorescence or internal heat conversion [27]. However, the singlet state PS may also convert to a triplet state via intersystem crossing, resulting in an electron spin change, which if reacted with molecular oxygen (as found in cells), it will give rise to free reactive oxygen species (ROS), which can result in tumor destruction [27].

Since the colon can be easily accessed via the rectum opening of the large intestine using an endoscope, this form of oncological PDT treatment for CRC tumors is possible [8]. Studies by Hodgkinson et al. [2] and Kawczyk-Krupta et al. [8] have noted that the PDT treatment of CRC which are inoperable, have only slightly advanced lesions/polyps or massive advanced tumors is a safe and feasible treatment option. Thus, colonoscopy endoscopes are used to directly deliver PS drugs to target tumor regions, as well as administer the required wavelength of laser irradiation light to activate a PS drug [2, 8].

The overall ability of PDT to successfully destroy cancer cells depends of the efficacy of ROS production in target cells. ROS can be produced via two different types of photoreactions (**Figure 2**) [26]. Within photoreaction type I, the PS drug reacts with surrounding cellular biomolecules via a hydrogen atom electron transfer to form free radicals, which react with cellular molecular oxygen, generating ROS, which in turn induces oxidative stress in target cells and so destroys them [27]. Whereby within photoreaction type II, the PS drug reacts directly with molecular oxygen in the cell to form singlet oxygen species, which are able to oxidize various substrates within target cells and so induce cell death [27]. When ROS and singlet oxygen species are generated from a PDT reaction, they are cytotoxic and so oxidize various substrates in a tumor cell inducing stress that triggers various cell death pathways such as apoptosis, autophagy or necrosis. Both types of photoreactions may occur simultaneously, however type I reactions generally favor apoptotic death in tumor cells [28]. Additionally, the effectivity of both photoreaction pathways depends on the type of

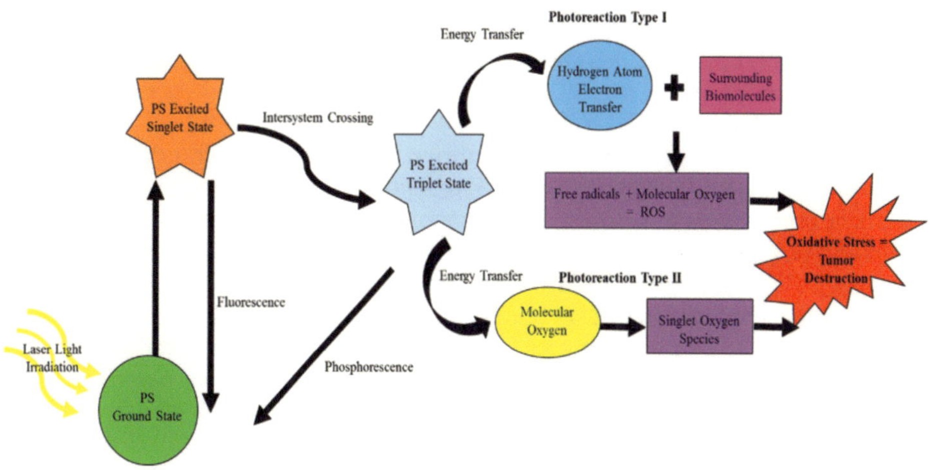

Figure 2.
PDT photophysical and photochemical mechanism of action for PS drug activation in tumor cells. When a PS drug is activated at a specific wavelength of light it becomes excited and so reacts with either molecular oxygen or other substrates within the surrounding areas of a cell, generating ROS, which in turn induces oxidative stress in cells triggering various cell death pathways and overall tumor destruction.

PS drug administered, where is localized in the tumor cell, as well as the amount of molecular oxygen present within the tumors microenvironment [29].

In the absence of laser irradiation light the PS drug remains inactive and so is not phototoxic in the body, therefore PDT can provide an alternative method to eradicate target tumor cells (since it is a localized treatment), while avoiding systematic toxicity and unwanted side effects when compared to conventional therapies (which affect healthy cells and tumor tissues) [26]. Thus, the major advantage of PDT over conventional therapies is that PS drugs tend to preferentially localize and be passively absorbed in tumor cells due to the enhanced permeability retention (EPR) effect and so their selective uptake can be achieved, allowing only minimal damage to healthy surrounding cells to occur during treatment [30]. Therefore, PDT can provide an alternative for the treatment of CRC, since it can avoid systematic toxicity, is minimally invasive, has a low morbidity rate, has the ability to preserve the anatomical function of healthy tissues, has minimal side effects, has no drug resistance and allows for repeated treatments [31].

However, in relation to PS drug delivery mechanisms CRC PDT research has now begun to focus on more selective passive (e.g. nanocarriers) and active (e.g. antigen–antibody targeting) uptake delivery mechanisms in tumor cells in order to further improve the efficacy of treatment [26]. These actively targeted PDT PS drug delivery mechanisms ensure preciously targeted PS drug delivery and localization in CRC only so that no damage occurs to normal healthy surrounding tissues [26].

4. PS drugs for CRC

PS drugs generate cytotoxic ROS or singlet oxygen species when they become activated at a particular wavelength, which in turn induces physical or chemical damage in target tumor cells [28]. In relation to the activation of PS drugs for effective PDT, it is important that they have a high molecular absorption coefficient within the red spectrum of light (650–780 nm), as to ensure maximum light absorption for PS excitation (as some endogenous human body pigments can absorb light), warrant minimal patient photosensitivity before treatment, as well as guarantee deep tissue penetration in target tumor sites [32, 33].

PSs are generally categorized into four different groups dependent on their functional capabilities. First generation PSs are one of the first types of PSs to be developed in PDT applications and they are stable, however have been shown to induce photosensitivity in patients and are activated within the lower red regions of light and so have a poor laser light tissue depth excitation range (e.g. haematoporphyrin derivatives) [33]. Second generation PSs have been further researched in PDT applications and since they are activated within the higher red regions of light, they have reported far less patient photosensitivity, with far deeper tissue laser light excitation (e.g. phthalocyanines, benzoporphyrins, purpurins, hypercin and chlorines [34]. Third generation PSs are currently the most promising PS drugs which are currently being researched within PDT cancer treatments [10]. Third generation PSs comprise of second generation PS drugs which have been chemically modified, functionalized or bound to nanoparticles (in order to promote their passive uptake) or active targeting biomolecules (such as aptamers, peptides, monoclonal antibodies, in order to promote their specific uptake in cancer cells only) [33]. In relation to current research, third generation PSs are reporting enhanced uptake in cancer cells with some of the most promising PDT treatment outcomes in CRC patients [33]. Lastly, most recent research has also begun to develop fourth-generation PS, which consist of second-generation PS encapsulated in a nanoparticle delivery system so its of third generation, however it is additionally co-encapsulated with a

Photosensitizer	Remarks	Ref.
***In vitro* PDT CRC research**		
3,4,5-trimethoxyphenyl, 3-hydroxyphenyl,4-hydroxyphenyl and sulfonamide phenyl porphyrin derivatives	Significant apoptotic cell death within HCT-116 CRC cells.	[37]
5,15-diaryltetrapyrrole derivatives porphyrin derivatives	Significant apoptotic cell death within HCT-116 CRC cells, with high yields of ROS being noted.	[38]
5-aminolevulinic acid	Enhanced PS uptake and improved PDT was noted within SW-480, HT-29 and CaCO-2 CRC cell lines.	[39]
5-aminolevulinic acid (ALA)	After PDT prognostic factor S100 protein concentration was reduced by 27% in SW480 and by 30% in SW620 CRC cell lines.	[40]
5-aminolevulinic acid (ALA)	Following PDT treatment autophagy cell death in human SW620 colon carcinoma cells was observed.	[41]
Chlorin e6 (Ce6)	CRC *in vitro* SW620 cells noted PDT induced apoptotic cell death.	[42]
Gallium phthalocyanine	CaCO-2 CRC cell line reported PDT induced cytotoxic effects.	[43]
Glycoconjugated chlorin (H2TFPC-SGlc)	MKN28, MKN45, HT29 and HCT116 CRC cell lines noted suppressed cell growth and apoptotic cell death post-PDT.	[44]
Hypericin	High doses induced massive ROS generation and severe ER stress, which then led apoptotic cell death while low doses triggered protective autophagy and promoted cell proliferation.	[45]
Indocyanine green	Effective ROS generation was observed with apoptotic cell death within *in vitro* cultured colon cancer cells at high PS concentrations.	[46]
Lysosome localizing Chlorin e6 (Ce6) ATX-S10Na(II)	Within CRC HCT116 cells, early apoptosis via Bax- and p53-dependent proteins was noted post-PDT.	[47]
Meta-tetra (hydroxyphenyl) chlorine (mTHPC)	Liposomal PS sub cellular localized localization in Colo-201 CRC cells was noted with significant cytotoxic apoptotic PDT induced cell death.	[48]
Meta-tetrahydroxyphenylchlorin	PS reported and effective PDT dose dependent effectivity in inhibiting cell proliferation, decreasing migration ability and colon formation within SW620 CRC cell lines.	[3]
Palmatine hydrochloride (PaH)	PDT showed significant photocytotoxicity on HT-29 cells and apoptotic cell death increased significantly in PS concentration-dependent and light dose-dependent manner.	[49]
Pheophorbide-a methyl ester (PPME)	HT-29 CRC cell line noted significant apoptotic cell death post-PDT treatment.	[50]
Photofrin II (Ph II) and hypericin (Hyp)	Combination of both PS post-PDT noted more effective cell death within doxorubicin-resistant LoVo DX CRC cell lines by reducing the multidrug resistance efflux protein P-glycoprotein (P-gp) and so promoted improved cytotoxic cell death.	[51]

Photosensitizer	Remarks	Ref.
Porfimer sodium (PII) and 2-[1-hexyloxyethyl]-2-devinylpyropheophorbide-a (HPPH)	PDT controlled metastatic tumor growth in murine colon 26-HA cells and enhanced anti tumor immunity.	[52]
Protoporphyrin IX (PpIX)	Enhanced the apoptosis in HCT116 CRC cell line	[53]
Sulfonated zinc phthalocyanine ($ZnPcS_{mix}$)	Within CRC DLD-1 and CaCo-2 cells the PS localized in multiple organelles and noted significant apoptotic PDT induced cell death.	[54]
Tetra-α-(4-carboxyphenoxy) phthalocyanine zinc	Noted interaction between p38 MAPK and caspase-9 regulated mitochondria-PDT mediated apoptosis in LoVo human colon carcinoma cells.	[55]
δ-aminolevulinic acid (ALA)	CRC cell lines SW480 and SW620 were treated in sublethal doses with ALA PDT in hypoxia-like conditions with cobalt chloride and noted decreases release of VEGF and significant tumor inhibition.	[56]
***In vivo* PDT CRC research**		
Bacteriochlorin analogues: 3-(1′-butyloxy) ethyl-3-deacetyl-bacteriopurpurin-18-N-butylimide methyl ester	High tumor uptake and long-term cure within BALB/c mice bearing Colon 26 tumors.	[57]
Hydrophilic bacteriochlorin (F2 BOH)	PDT enabled long-term cures of BALB/c mice with subcutaneously implanted CT26 tumors, and the cured mice rejected tumor re-inoculation 1 year after the treatment.	[58]
Metalloporphyrin Ga-4cisPtTPyP (5,10,15,20-tetrakis{cis-diammine-chloro-platinum(II)}(4-pyridyl)-porphyrinato gallium(III) hydroxide tetranitrate)	High tumor accumulation and almost completely inhibited tumor growth over 2 weeks in BALB/c mice bearing Colon 26 tumors.	[59]
Photosan-II (PS-II) and chloroquine	Significantly reduced the tumor size in a xenograft mice model and induced apoptotic and autophagy cell death within *in vitro* SW620 and HCT116 cells.	[60]
Porphyrazine platform with gadolinium (III) cation chelated by tetrapyrrole macrocycles (GdPz1 and GdPz2)	Selective *in vivo* accumulation within murine colon carcinoma CT26 models was observed, with significant inhibition of tumor growth.	[61]
Redaporfin	Single dose was well tolerated by male BALB/c mice with subcutaneously implanted colon (CT26) tumors and PDT led to the complete tumor regression in 83% of the mice.	[62]

Table 1.
Current PDT studies which utilize different types of PS for the in vitro, in vivo or clinical treatment of CRC.

small-molecular inhibitor system capable of blocking any tumor survival pathways post PDT, in order to halt possible tumor reoccurrence [35]. However, in relation to fourth-generation PSS this form of PDT treatment research is limited to only being able to target and inhibit VEGFs, in order to promote PS drugs uptake and so deter the neovascularization of tumors, preventing CRC tumor metastatic spread and reoccurrence [35].

At the moment clinically FDA approved first and second generation PSs for PDT oncology include: Porfimer sodium (Photofrin), 5-Aminolevulinic acid

(Levulan), Methyl aminolevulinate (Metvixia), Meta tetra(hydroxyphenyl) chlorin (Foscan), N-aspartyl chlorin e6 (NPe6, Laserphyrin), Benzoporphyrin derivative monoacid ring A (Visudyne) and N-hexyl ester of ALA (Cysview) [32–35]. Whereas, first- and second-generation PSs, which are currently under clinical trials include; Hypocrellin A, Pheophorbide-a, Chlorin e6, Methylene Blue, Hypericin, Phthalocyanine, Rose Bengal, HPPH: 2-(1-Hexyl-oxyethyl)-2-devinyl pyropheophorbide-alpha [30, 34, 36]. However, in relation to third and fourth generation PSs, none to date have received clinical approval for PDT CRC treatments and so remain a commanding area of research focus [26]. **Table 1** shows various research studies currently that have been performed with different types of PSs for the PDT treatment of CRC.

To date only one single successful clinical study from 2016, utilizing Photofrin II (Ph II) PS PDT drug on 23 young patients with advanced CRC, noted improved clinical symptoms and reduce complications post-PDT treatment [63]. These findings suggest that more research is required to develop better PS drugs to withstand clinical trials.

5. PDT CRC clinical challenges

Despite the many positive features of CRC PDT, within clinical settings this form of treatment has experienced some drawbacks in relation to PS drug solubility, mode of delivery and selective tumor uptake [64, 65].

In order to ensure the maximum levels of ROS are generated during a PDT treatment, as to ensure complete tumor destruction, the highest possible concentrations of PS drugs must be able to be successfully delivered and localize in target tumor tissues [27]. Within PDT clinical settings using first and second generation PS drugs, poor outcomes and effectiveness has been noted, as only minor amounts of PS drugs are able to overcome the human bodies biological barriers and so passively accumulate (due to the EPR effect) in tumor cells, generating very low levels ROS and tumor destruction [2, 31]. Additionally, due to this passivation process sometimes PS drugs can accumulate in healthy tissues inducing unwanted PDT side effects such as patients' photosensitivity and damage to normal tissues [26].

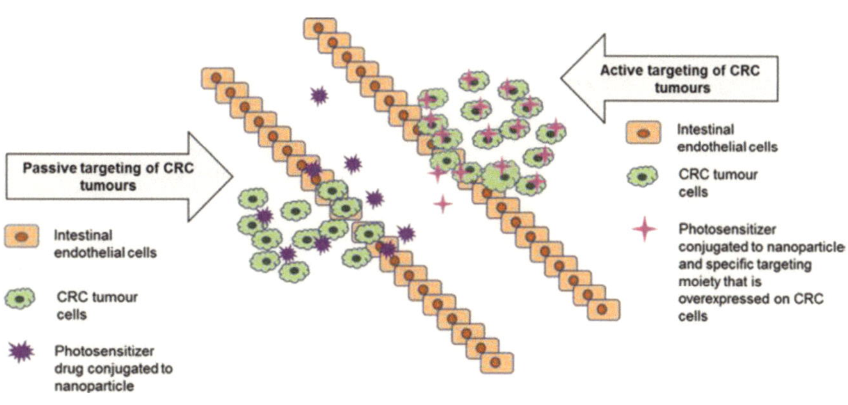

Figure 3.
Passive PS NP drug delivery versus active targeting moiety conjugated PS NP drug delivery, which shows targeted and enhanced CRC tumor PS drug uptake for more effective PDT treatment outcomes.

Another issue sometimes noted in clinical settings is that PS drugs have limited solubility and so tend to aggregate during administration, limiting their overall uptake and effectivity [2]. Moreover, a PS drugs concentrated subcellular localization in a tumors mitochondria, lysosomes, endoplasmic reticulum, plasma membrane etc., is of utmost importance since ROS have only a very short half-life and so will only induce effective cell death in tumor cells if they are proximately localized within these organelles [29, 32].

Thus, shortcomings such as poor solubility, bioavailability, maximum ROS generation and tumor subcellular localization targeting need to be overcome in order to ensure the effectivity of PDT [26]. Nevertheless third generation PS drug nanoparticle (NP) drug carriers are currently being investigated to ensure PS drug solubility and improved passive uptake, with functionalized active targeting abilities (e.g. overexpressed peptides), as to ensure specific uptake in tumor cells only to enhance the overall efficacy of PDT (**Figure 3**) [29, 32].

6. Nanoparticles for enhanced passive PS drug delivery and PDT

Passive PS uptake makes use of the drugs physiochemical factors, as well as the morphological and physiological differences between tumor and tissues (i.e. EPR effect) to allow PSs to accumulate in tumor sites [30].

There has been great interest in combining PS drugs with NPs in order to overcome some of the challenges conventional PS drug delivery mechanisms experience in clinical settings [65]. This is because NPs can enhance PS drug passive uptake, promote solubility, stability and limit non-specific toxicity [66]. Additionally, NPs can mimic biological molecules and so when combined with PSs, they go by unnoticed by immune barriers, remaining in tacked and so improved passivation of PS drug uptake in tumors [33]. Examples of nanoparticle platforms to assist in the passivation PS drug delivery for PDT CRC treatment include: liposomes, polymers, micelles, dendrimers, silica, nanoemulsion, nanotubes and nanogels [67]. Moreover, these NP platforms (especially polymeric NPs) have the additional benefit of protecting PS drugs against chemical and enzymatic gastrointestinal tract degradation, and so increase the drugs stability and cellular uptake within the intestinal epithelium [68, 69]. Various studies listing the effective passive PS drug delivery in CRC tumors utilizing NP carrier platforms have been listed in **Table 2**.

***In vitro* and *in vivo* PDT CRC research**			
Photosensitizer	**Nanoparticle**	**Remarks**	**Ref.**
5-(4-aminophenyl)-10,15,20-triphenylchlorin and 5-(4-carboxyphenyl)-10,15,20-triphenylchlorin	Chitosan	Drugs localized in endocytic vesicles of HCT116/LUC human colon carcinoma cells and within tumor-bearing mice, showed strong PDT treatment.	[70]
5,10,15,20-Tetrakis(4-hydroxy-phenyl)-21H, 23H-porphine (pTHPP)	Polyhydroxyalkanoates (PHAs)	*In vitro* photocytotoxicity in human colon adenocarcinoma cell line HT-29 revealed time and concentration dependent cell death.	[71]
5-aminolevulinic acid	Co polymer methoxy poly(ethylene glycol)-chitosan	Enhanced delivery and PDT phototoxicity.	[72]
5-aminolevulinic acid (ALA)	Chitosan	Enhanced cellular absorption in Caco-2CRC cells.	[73]
5-flurouraci (5-FU)	Solid lipid	Enhanced delivery and PDT phototoxicity, within CRC cells and chemo resistant stem-like cells.	[74]

***In vitro* and *in vivo* PDT CRC research**			
Photosensitizer	**Nanoparticle**	**Remarks**	**Ref.**
Chlorin e6 (Ce6)	Methoxy poly(ethylene glycol) (MePEG)	Showed enhanced cellular uptake, phototoxicity, and ROS generation within *in vitro* CRC cells and reported improved tumor tissue penetration and accumulation within *in vivo* animal studies.	[75]
Chlorin e6 (Ce6)	Polymeric carrier polyvinyl alcohol (PVA)	Noted higher uptake in murine colon carcinoma CT26 tumors models with significant tumor regression and necrotic cell death.	[76]
Chlorin e6 (Ce6)	Doxorubicin (DOX)-loaded micelles with mPEG lipoic acid (LA)	PS and anticancer drug are colocalized in within *in vitro* CT-26 and HCT-116 CRC cells. Dual therapy induced apoptotic cell death and inhibited tumor growth in CT-26 tumor bearing mouse model	[77]
Curcumin and 5-fluorouracil	Chitosan	CRC HT29 cell line had a 3-fold increase in anticancer effects.	[78]
Cyanine IR-780	Solid lipid and flavonoid derivatives for electroporation	Showed improved uptake and demonstrated the ability to act as an anticancer PDT modality to eliminate LoVo and CHO-K1 CRC cells in vitro	[79]
Diaryl-porphyrin (PMMA@ PorVa)	Core-shell poly-methyl methacrylate	Human colon carcinoma cell line HCT116 noted PDT induced apoptotic cell death.	[80]
Dimeric zinc(II) phthalocyanine	Alkyne-modified mesoporous silica	Exhibited high intracellular fluorescence in human colon adenocarcinoma HT29 cells with notable photocytotoxicity	[81]
Hypericin	Pluronic P123 (P123)	*In vitro* Caco-2 and HT-29 intestinal colon carcinoma cells noted 90% photocytotoxic cell death.	[82]
Indocyanine green (icg)	Super carbonate apatite (sCA)	*In vitro* and *in vivo* HT29 CRC tumors exhibited drastic and highly significant tumor growth retardation.	[83]
IR780 iodide	Pluronic coated gold	Show enhanced phototherapeutic and photothermal activity with no dark cytotoxicity within *in vitro* murine colon carcinoma cells (C26).	[84]
Meso-tetra (carboxyphenyl) porphyrin (TCPP)	Poly(D,L-lactide-*co*-glycolide) (PLGA)	Improved uptake of PS, with enhanced phototoxicity within *in vitro* SW480CRC cells and dramatic tumor-inhibiting efficacy in four-week-old female athymic mice.	[16]
Meta-tetra (hydroxyphenyl) chlorine (mTHPC)	Liposomal formulation FosPeg®	Improved PS absorption with enhanced phototoxicity and cell death in HT29 cell lines.	[85]
Oxaliplatin	Chitosan micelles	Eliminated bulk CRC cell populations and stem-like cells both *in vitro* and *in vivo*.	[86]
Photoprotoporphyrin IX dimethyl ester (PppIX-DME)	Polyethylene glycol and polylactic acid block copolymer (PN-Por)	Noted improved uptake and sustained release within *in vitro* Colon-26 carcinoma and efficient tumor deposition was found in C26 tumor-bearing mice with a significant and highly effective PDT anti-tumor effect.	[87]
Porfimer sodium (PII) and 2-[1-hexyloxyethyl]-2-devinylpyropheophorbide-a (HPPH)	Polymeric tubule-forming phospholipid, DC PC with PEGylated lipid	Enhanced tumor accumulation and superior therapeutic efficacy in HT29 tumor mouse xenographs and Colon-26 bearing BALB/c mice showed no tumor reoccurrence up to 100 days.	[88]
Porphyrin	Nano micelles and SN-38 (7-ethyl-10-hydroxycamptothecin) chemotherapeutic drug	Synergistic chemo drug and PS dramatically enhanced *in vivo* antitumor PDT efficacy over single treatment in nude mice bearing HT-29 colon cancer xenograft.	[89]

In vitro and *in vivo* PDT CRC research			
Photosensitizer	**Nanoparticle**	**Remarks**	**Ref.**
Protoporphyrin IX (PpIX)	Non-biodegradable silica	Improved PS accumulation in both HCT-116 cell lines and tumor bearing mice, with enhanced ROS generation.	[90]
SN-38-Cyclodextrin Complexation	Chlorin-core star-shaped block copolymer (CSBC) micelles	Combination of PS and chemotherapy nanocarrier showed 60% tumor regression in HT-29 human CRC xenograft model, after three applications.	[91]
Zinc phthalocyanine	Liposomal	CRC CT26 tumor models which received PDT and sonodynamic therapy tumors shrank by 20% after 120 days.	[92]
Zinc phthalocyanine	Titanium dioxide	Improved uptake and enhanced theranostics of PDT within *in vitro* colorectal adenocarcinoma (HT29) cells.	[93]
Zinc protoporphyrin (ZnPP)	N-(2-hydroxypropyl) methacrylamide copolymer with PEG	Nanodrug caused necrosis and disappearance of >70% of tumors in colon cancer mouse models.	[94]
Zinc(II) phthalocyanine	Tetronic® 1107 polymeric poloxamine micelles (T1107)	Improved uptake and enhanced PDT apoptotic cell death within *in vitro* 2D and 3D murine colon adenocarcinoma CT26 cells.	[95]

Table 2.
Passive Targeting PDT PS drug delivery mechanisms within in vitro and in vivo CRC.

7. Active targeting biomolecules for enhanced PS drug delivery and PDT

Active PDT PS drug delivery involves the conjugation of the PS drug to specific ligands or biomolecules moieties, which are complementary to overexpressed cancer cell receptors and so via a molecular recognition process PS drug uptake in target tumor cells is enhanced [31]. These moieties include monoclonal antibodies (mAb), proteins (e.g. transferrin), nucleic acids (aptamers), small molecules (folic acid), polymers (hyaluronic acid) and peptides (proteins), which are over-expressed on CRC tumor cells only [31, 96]. These specific ligands or biomolecules moieties, which are conjugated to a PS NP drug delivery system, have a specific affinity for receptors that are over-expressed on CRC tumor cells and their vascular, but not on normal cells [34]. This facilitates enhanced PSs retention in tumor target sites only, improving the efficacy of PDT and localizing its treatments effectiveness to killing CRC tumors only [34]. Common protein receptors in CRC cells which have been noted to be overexpressed and so can be utilized for possible PS active drug targeting include: epidermal growth factor receptor (EGFR), fibroblast growth factor receptor (FGFR), epithelial cell-adhesion molecule (EpCAM), carbonic anhydrase IX (CA IX), peroxisome proliferator-activated receptor γ (PPARγ), cyclooxygenase-2 (COX-2), cholesterol and low-density lipoprotein, estrogen receptors, cholecystokinin A receptors, lectin saccharide receptors, anti-DR5 antibody, as well as cluster of differentiation 44, 133, 166 and 24 (CD44+, CD 133+, CD166+ and CD24+) [13, 97–99]. Recent research approaches to enhance PS NP drug delivery by actively targeting CRC tumors using various moieties and so increase the efficacy of PDT have been listed in **Table 3**.

***In vitro* and *in vivo* PDT CRC research**			
Photosensitizer	**Active drug delivery system**	**Remarks**	**Ref.**
5-Fluorouracil	Eudragit S100 coated citrus pectin nanoparticles	Eudragit S100 is a pH responsive enteric polymer and citrus pectin is a ligand receptor for galectin-3. Targeted drug delivery was found both *in vitro* and *in vivo* with enhanced PDT cytotoxic effects.	[100]
Chlorin e6 (Ce6)	Site specific immune-conjugates (murine monoclonal antibody 17.1A)	Cationic electric charge of photoimmune-conjugate enhanced PS delivery and showed a 90% phototoxic effect within *in vitro* HT-29CRC cells.	[46]
Chlorin e6 (Ce6)	Phototoxic DNA aptamers were bound to unique short O-glycan-peptide signatures	Drug conjugate reported >500-fold increase in toxicity upon light activation in HT-29CRC cells and was not cytotoxic towards cell types without O-glycan-peptide markers.	[101]
Chlorin e6 (Ce6) and indium	Biotinylated to target biotin receptors	Colon carcinoma *in vitro* CT26 cell lines showed targeted uptake with enhanced apoptotic cell death.	[102]
Chlorin e6 (Ce6)	Hyaluronic acid conjugated to 5β-cholanic acid (5β-CA) to target CD44 ligands	Effective tumor targeting noted with tumor growth being significantly suppressed and inhibited by 9.61 ± 1.09-fold in human colon HT29 cell line and murine tumor model.	[103]
Chlorin e6 (Ce6)	Hyaluronic acid nanoparticle to target CD 44 receptors	Enhanced uptake in human colon cancer xenograft model was observed with significant tumor destruction.	[104]
Chlorin e6 (Ce6)	Glycoconjugated chlorin (G-chlorin)	PDT induced significant targeted immunogenic apoptotic cell death in a syngeneic CT26 mouse tumor model (allograft model)	[105]
Hypericin	Histone deacetylase inhibitor sodium phenylbutyrate (NaPB)	Reported significant increase in tumor suppressor CDKN1A gene in CRC model with enhanced uptake and PDT effects.	[106]
IR780 iodide	Self-assembled transferrin-IR780 for direct Transferrin-receptor (TfR) targeting	Within Murine CT26 colon carcinoma cells and CT26 tumor-bearing mice notable targeting and tumor suppression was observed.	[107]
Meso-tetraphenyl chlorin disulfonate (TPCS2a)	IM7-saporin immunotoxin CD44 targeting receptor	Drug carrier was successfully transported into *in vitro* WiDr CRC cells via photochemical internalization (PCI) and resulted in 90% cytotoxic response.	[108]
Meta-tetra(hydroxyphenyl) chlorin (mTHPC)	Bevacizumab (Avastin™), an anti-VEGF neutralizing monoclonal antibody	PDT PS with Avastin™ and monoclonal antibody in murine model, reported even lowered expression of VEGF in tumors with improved tumor killing efficacy than when compared to anti-angiogenic chemotherapeutic Avastin™ and monoclonal antibody treatment alone (which indirectly kills cells by via vascular damage), suggesting that PDT PS contributed to overall combined treatment approach by directly killing cells via ROS generation as well, and so improved CRC cell death.	[109]
None	Photothermal gold coated superparamagnetic iron oxide nanoparticles conjugated with thiol modified MUC-1 aptamers	Photothermal therapy of colon cancer cells exhibited notable cell death.	[110]

In vitro and *in vivo* PDT CRC research			
Photosensitizer	**Active drug delivery system**	**Remarks**	**Ref.**
Pyropheophorbide-a (PPa) protoporphyrin	ATP-binding cassette subfamily G2 (ABCG2) porphyrin-based targeted PDT.	PS drug delivery was improved within *in vitro* HT29 cells show high levels of ABCG2 expression with significant PDT induced cell damage.	[111]
Pyropheophorbide-a methyl ester (PPME)	Peroxisomal proliferator-activated receptor gamma (PPARγ) ligand troglitazone	Enhanced uptake in DLD-1 CRC *in vitro* cells, with significant growth retardation and apoptotic cell death in a PDT dose-dependent manner.	[112]
Verteporfin succinimidyl ester	Single chain variable fragments (scFvs), antibody fragments	Improved uptake and within *in vitro* and *in vivo* PDT applications it effectively killed tumor LoVo (CEA+, HER2-) cells.	[44]
Zinc phthalocyanine (C11Pc)	HER2 receptor or jacalin, a lectin specific for carbohydrate T antigen on PEG Gold nanoparticles	HT-29 CRC cells reported enhanced targeted PDT with 80–90% cell death being noted.	[113]

Table 3.
Active Targeting PDT PS drug delivery mechanisms within in vitro and in vivo CRC.

8. Conclusion

From this chapter it can be observed that PDT is most definitely a highly effective and alternative therapeutic treatment for CRC [8]. However, conventional PS drug delivery applications have numerous limitations in relation to solubility and poor tumor subcellular localization specificity [26]. Nevertheless, NP PS drug delivery systems which are surface functionalized with various tumor-targeting moieties can help overcoming some of these limitations be passively, as well as actively enhancing PS drug uptake.

In this chapter, we have shown that there are many positive and promising research studies being conducted *in vitro* and *in vivo*, for the use of PDT in CRC treatment (**Table 1**). We have also evidenced the remarkable potential of passivation NP PS drug carrier platforms (**Table 2**) and specific receptor based PS drug active targeting (**Table 3**), in order to promote the selective absorption of PS drugs in target CRC tumor sites only and so avoid unwanted side effects, as well as overall enhance the PDT treatment of CRC. However, it must be noted that the research studies which have been reported in **Tables 2** and **3** are within early stages of *in vitro* and *in vivo* research and no clinical trials have been performed as of yet. Thus, researchers need to start further exploring specific functionalized NP PS drug delivery platforms for the targeted drug delivery of PSs and effective PDT treatment of CRC within pre-clinical and clinical trials in order to develop optimized standards for this form of CRC therapy [8]. The findings from these studies should drive the application of targeted PDT PS drug delivery to the forefront of oncological interventions as a possible treatment modality for the eradication of CRC.

Acknowledgements

The authors sincerely thank the University of Johannesburg, South African Research Chairs Initiative of the Department of Science and Technology and

National Research Foundation of South Africa (Grant No 98337), National Research Foundation Thuthuka Fund (Grant No TTK180409318735) and Cancer Association of South Africa (CANSA) Research Funding Grant for their financial grant support.

Conflict of interest

The authors confirm that this chapter has no conflict of interest.

Author details

Cherie Ann Kruger and Heidi Abrahamse*
Faculty of Health Sciences, Laser Research Centre, University of Johannesburg, South Africa

*Address all correspondence to: habrahamse@uj.ac.za

References

[1] Mármol I, Sánchez-de-Diego C, Pradilla Dieste A, et al. Colorectal carcinoma: A general overview and future perspectives in colorectal cancer. International Journal of Molecular Sciences. 2017;**18**(1):E197. DOI: 10.3390/ijms18010197

[2] Hodgkinson N, Kruger CA, Abrahamse H. Targeted photodynamic therapy as potential treatment modality for the eradication of colon cancer and colon cancer stem cells. Tumor Biology. 2017;**39**(10):1010428317734691. DOI: 10.1177/1010428317734691

[3] Abdulrehman G, Xv K, Li Y, Kang L. Effects of meta-tetrahydroxyphenylchlorin photodynamic therapy on isogenic colorectal cancer SW480 and SW620 cells with different metastatic potentials. Lasers in Medical Science. 2018;**33**:1581-1590. DOI: 10.1007/s10103-018-2524-7

[4] Bogaert J, Prenen H. Molecular genetics of colorectal cancer. Annals of Gastroenterology. 2014;**27**(1):9-14

[5] Palaghia M, Prelipcean CC, Cotea E, et al. Metastatic colorectal cancer: Review of diagnosis and treatment options. Journal of Surgery. 2015;**10**(4):249-256. DOI: 10.7438/1584-9341-10-4-2

[6] Garza-Treviño EN, Said-Fernández SL, Martínez-Rodríguez HG. Understanding the colon cancer stem cells and perspectives on treatment. Cancer Cell International. 2015;**15**(1):2. DOI: 10.1186/s12935-015-0163-7

[7] Huiskens J, van Gulik TM, van Lienden KP, et al. Treatment strategies in colorectal cancer patients with initially unresectable liver-only metastases, a study protocol of the randomised phase 3 CAIRO5 study of the dutch colorectal cancer group (DCCG). BMC Cancer. 2015;**15**(1):365. DOI: 10.1186/s12885-015-1323-9

[8] Kawczyk-Krupka A, Bugaj AM, Latos W, et al. Photodynamic therapy in colorectal cancer treatment: The state of the art in clinical trials. Photodiagnosis and Photodynamic Therapy. 2015;**12**(3):545-553. DOI: 10.1016/j.pdpdt.2015.04.004

[9] Xu R, Zhou B, Fung PCW, et al. Recent advances in the treatment of colon cancer. Histology and Histopathology. 2006;**21**(8):867-872. DOI: 10.14670/HH-21.867

[10] Hagan S, Orr MC, Doyle B. Targeted therapies in colorectal cancer—An integrative view by PPPM. The EPMA Journal. 2013;**4**(1):3. DOI: 10.1186/1878-5085-4-3

[11] Schwartz RN, Blanke CD. Targeted therapies in the treatment of colorectal cancer: What managed care needs to know. Journal of Managed Care Pharmacy. 2004;**10**(5 suppl B):S2-S13

[12] McKeown E, Nelson DW, Johnson EK, et al. Current approaches and challenges for monitoring treatment response in colon and rectal cancer. Journal of Cancer. 2014;**5**(1):31-43. DOI: 10.7150/jca.7987

[13] Treating Colorectal Cancer [Internet]. 2018. Available from: https://www.cancer.org/cancer/colon-rectal-cancer/treating/by-stage-colon.html [Accessed: Jan 24, 2019]

[14] Van der Jeught K, Xu H, Li Y, et al. Drug resistance and new therapies in colorectal cancer. World Journal of Gastroenterology. 2018;**24**(34):3834-3848. DOI: 10.3748/wjg.v24.i34.3834

[15] Falchook GS, Kurzrock R. VEGF and dual-EGFR inhibition

in colorectal cancer. Cell Cycle. 2015;**14**(8):1129-1130. DOI: 10.1080/15384101.2015.1022071

[16] Hu Z, Pan Y, Wang J, et al. Meso-tetra (carboxyphenyl) porphyrin (TCPP) nanoparticles were internalized by SW480 cells by a clathrin-mediated endocytosis pathway to induce high photocytotoxicity. Biomedicine & Pharmacotherapy. 2009;**63**:155-164. DOI: 10.1016/j.biopha.2008.07.087

[17] Constant S, Huang S, Wiszniewski L, et al. Colon cancer: Current treatments and preclinical models for the discovery and development of new therapies. In: El-Shemy HA, editor. Drug Discovery. Rijeka: IntechOpen; 2013. DOI: 10.5772/53391

[18] Lin C, Ng HL, Pan W, et al. Exploring different strategies for efficient delivery of colorectal cancer therapy. International Journal of Molecular Sciences. 2015;**16**:26936-26952. DOI: 10.3390/ijms161125995

[19] Hammond WA, Swaika A, Mody K. Pharmacologic resistance in colorectal cancer: A review. Therapeutic Advances in Medical Oncology. 2016;**8**(1):57-84. DOI: 10.1177/1758834015614530

[20] Willett CG, Duda DG, Czito BG, et al. Targeted therapy in rectal cancer. Oncology. 2007;**21**(9):1055-1065

[21] Thomas J, Beinhorn C, Norton D, et al. Managing radiation therapy side effects with complementary medicine. Journal of the Society for Integrative Oncology. 2010;**8**(2):65-80

[22] Jin H, Gao S, Guo H, et al. Re-sensitization of radiation resistant colorectal cancer cells to radiation through inhibition of AMPK pathway. Oncology Letters. 2016;**11**(5):3197-3201. DOI: 10.3892/ol.2016.4339

[23] Geng L, Wang J. Molecular effectors of radiation resistance in colorectal cancer. Precision Radiation Oncology. 2017;**1**:27-33. DOI: 10.1002/pro6.5

[24] Anderson EC, Hessman C, Levin TG, et al. The role of colorectal cancer stem cells in metastatic disease and therapeutic response. Cancers. 2011;**3**(1):319-339. DOI: 10.3390/cancers3010319

[25] DeSantis CE, Lin CC, Mariotto AB, et al. Cancer treatment and survivorship statistics, 2014. CA: A Cancer Journal for Clinicians. 2014;**64**(4):252-271. DOI: 10.3322/caac.21235

[26] Kruger CA, Abrahamse H. Utilisation of targeted nanoparticle photosensitiser drug delivery systems for the enhancement of photodynamic therapy. Molecules. 2018;**23**:2628. DOI: 10.3390/molecules23102628

[27] Baptista MS, Cadet J, Di Mascio P, et al. Type I and II photosensitized oxidation reactions: Guidelines and mechanistic pathways. Photochemistry and Photobiology. 2017;**93**(4):912-919. DOI: 10.1111/php.12716

[28] Hu Z, Oleinick N, Hamblin MR. Photodynamic therapy as an emerging treatment modality for cancer and non-cancer diseases. Journal of Analytical and Bioanalytical Techniques. 2014;**S1**:e001. DOI: 10.4172/2155-9872.S1-e001

[29] Abrahamse H, Hamblin MR. New photosensitizers for photodynamic therapy. The Biochemical Journal. 2016;**473**(4):347-364. DOI: 10.1042/BJ20150942

[30] Yoo JO, Ha KS. New insights into the mechanisms for photodynamic therapy-induced cancer cell death. International Review of Cell and Molecular Biology. 2012;**295**:139-174. DOI: 10.1016/B978-0-12-394306-4.00010-1

[31] Olivo M, Bhuvaneswari R, Lucky SS, et al. Targeted therapy of cancer using photodynamic therapy in combination with multi-faceted anti-tumor modalities. Pharmaceuticals. 2010;**3**(5):1507-1529. DOI: 10.3390/ph3051507

[32] Chen G, Roy I, Yang C, et al. Nanochemistry and nanomedicine for nanoparticle-based diagnostics and therapy. Chemical Reviews. 2016;**116**(5):2826-2885. DOI: 10.1021/acs.chemrev.5b00148

[33] Debele TA, Peng S, Tsai HC. Drug carrier for photodynamic cancer therapy. International Journal of Molecular Sciences. 2015;**16**(9):22094-22136. DOI: 10.3390/ijms160922094

[34] Zhang J, Jiang C, Longo JPF, et al. An updated overview on the development of new photosensitizers for anticancer photodynamic therapy. Acta Pharmaceutica Sinica B. 2018;**8**(2):137-146. DOI: 10.1016/j.apsb.2017.09.003

[35] Kataoka H, Nishie H, Hayashi N, et al. New photodynamic therapy with next-generation photosensitizers. Annals of Translational Medicine. 2017;**5**(8):183. DOI: 10.21037/atm.2017.03.59

[36] Calixto GM, Bernegossi J, de Freitas LM, et al. Nanotechnology-based drug delivery systems for photodynamic therapy of cancer: A review. Molecules. 2016;**21**(3):342. DOI: 10.3390/molecules21030342

[37] Banfi S, Caruso E, Caprioli S, et al. Photodynamic effects of porphyrin and chlorin photosensitizers in human colon adenocarcinoma cells. Bioorganic & Medicinal Chemistry. 2004;**12**(18):4853-4860. DOI: 10.1016/j.bmc.2004.07.011

[38] Gariboldi MB, Ravizza R, Baranyai P, et al. Photodynamic effects of novel 5,15-diaryl-tetrapyrrole derivatives on human colon carcinoma cells. Bioorganic & Medicinal Chemistry. 2009;**17**(5):2009-2016. DOI: 10.1016/j.bmc.2009.01.035

[39] Brunner H, Hausmann F, Krieg RC, et al. The effects of 5-aminolevulinic acid esters on protoporphyrin IX production in human adenocarcinoma cell lines. Photochemistry and Photobiology. 2001;**74**(5):721-725

[40] Kawczyk-Krupka A, Latos W, Latos M, et al. ALA-induced photodynamic effect on viability, apoptosis and secretion of S100 protein, secreted by colon cancer cells in vitro. Photodiagnosis and Photodynamic Therapy. 2016;**15**:218-227. DOI: 10.1016/j.pdpdt.2016.07.009

[41] Ziółkowska B, Woźniak M, Ziółkowski P. Co-expression of autophagic markers following photodynamic therapy in SW620 human colon adenocarcinoma cells. Molecular Medicine Reports. 2016;**14**(3):2548-2554. DOI: 10.3892/mmr.2016.5541

[42] Yang K, Niu T, Luo M, et al. Enhanced cytotoxicity and apoptosis through inhibiting autophagy in metastatic potential colon cancer SW620 cells treated with Chlorin e6 photodynamic therapy. Photodiagnosis and Photodynamic Therapy. 2018;**24**:332-341. DOI: 10.1016/j.pdpdt.2018.10.012

[43] Maduray K, Odhav B. Efficacy of gallium phthalocyanine as a photosensitizing agent in photodynamic therapy for the treatment of cancer. In: Proceedings of the SPIE 8553: Optics in Health Care and Biomedical Optics V/COS Photonics Asia, Beijing, China. Vol. 85530G. Bellingham, WA: SPIE; 2012

[44] Tanaka M, Kataoka H, Mabuchi M, et al. Anticancer effects of novel photodynamic therapy with glycoconjugated chlorin for gastric and

colon cancer. Anticancer Research. 2011;**31**(3):763-769

[45] Lin S, Yang L, Shi H, et al. Endoplasmic reticulum-targeting photosensitizer hypericin confers chemo-sensitization towards oxaliplatin through inducing pro-death autophagy. The International Journal of Biochemistry & Cell Biology. 2017;**87**:54-68. DOI: 10.1016/j.biocel.2017.04.001

[46] Ruhi MK, AK A, Gülsoy M. Dose-dependent photochemical/photothermal toxicity of indocyanine green-based therapy on three different cancer cell lines. Photodiagnosis and Photodynamic Therapy. 2018;**21**:334-343. DOI: 10.1016/j.pdpdt.2018.01.008

[47] Mitsunaga M, Tsubota A, Nariai K, et al. Early apoptosis and cell death induced by ATX-S10Na (II)-mediated photodynamic therapy are Bax- and p53-dependent in human colon cancer cells. World Journal of Gastroenterology. 2007;**13**(5):692-698

[48] Leung WN, Sun X, Mak NK, et al. Photodynamic effects of mTHPC on human colon adenocarcinoma cells: Photocytotoxicity, subcellular localization and apoptosis. Photochemistry and Photobiology. 2002;**75**(4):406-411

[49] Wu J, Xiao Q, Zhang N, et al. Photodynamic action of palmatine hydrochloride on colon adenocarcinoma HT-29 cells. Photodiagnosis and Photodynamic Therapy. 2016;**15**:53-58. DOI: 10.1016/j.pdpdt.2016.05.005

[50] Xu CS, Leung AWN, Liu L, et al. LED-activated pheophorbide a induces cellular destruction of colon cancer cells. Laser Physics Letters. 2010;7(7):544-548. DOI: 10.1002/lapl.201010008

[51] Saczko J, Kulbacka J, Chwilkowska A, et al. Cytosolic superoxide dismutase activity after photodynamic therapy, intracellular distribution of Photofrin II and hypericin, and P-glycoprotein localization in human colon adenocarcinoma. Folia Histochemica et Cytobiologica. 2007;**45**(2):93-98

[52] Shams M, Owczarczak B, Manderscheid-Kern P, et al. Development of photodynamic therapy regimens that control primary tumor growth and inhibit secondary disease. Cancer Immunology, Immunotherapy. 2015;**64**(3):287-297. DOI: 10.1007/s00262-014-1633-9

[53] Ouyang G, Liu Z, Xiong L, et al. Role of PpIX-based photodynamic therapy in promoting the damage and apoptosis of colorectal cancer cell and its mechanisms. Journal of Central South University. Medical sciences. 2017;**42**(8):874-881. DOI: 10.11817/j.issn.1672-7347.2017.08.002

[54] Sekhejane PR, Houreld NN, Abrahamse H. Multiorganelle localization of metallated phthalocyanine photosensitizer in colorectal cancer cells (DLD-1 and CaCo-2) enhances efficacy of photodynamic therapy. International Journal of Photoenergy. 2014;**383027**:10. DOI: 10.1155/2014/383027

[55] Wang Y, Xia C, Lun Z, et al. Crosstalk between p38 MAPK and caspase-9 regulates mitochondria-mediated apoptosis induced by tetra-α-(4-carboxyphenoxy) phthalocyanine zinc photodynamic therapy in LoVo cells. Oncology Reports. 2018;**39**(1):61-70. DOI: 10.3892/or.2017.6071

[56] Kawczyk-Krupka A, Kwiatek B, Czuba ZP, et al. Secretion of the angiogenic factor VEGF after photodynamic therapy with ALA under hypoxia-like conditions in colon cancer cells. Photodiagnosis and Photodynamic Therapy. 2018;**21**:16-18. DOI: 10.1016/j.pdpdt.2017.10.020

[57] Patel N, Pera P, Joshi P, et al. Highly effective dual-function near-infrared (NIR) photosensitizer for fluorescence imaging and photodynamic therapy (PDT) of cancer. Journal of Medicinal Chemistry. 2016;**59**(21):9774-9787. DOI: 10.1021/acs.jmedchem.6b00890

[58] Luz AFS, Pucelik B, Pereira MM, et al. Translating phototherapeutic indices from in vitro to in vivo photodynamic therapy with bacteriochlorins. Lasers in Surgery and Medicine. 2018;**50**(5):451-459. DOI: 10.1002/lsm.22931

[59] Hu X, Ogawa K, Kiwada T, et al. Water-soluble metalloporphyrinates with excellent photo-induced anticancer activity resulting from high tumor accumulation. Journal of Inorganic Biochemistry. 2017;**170**:1-7. DOI: 10.1016/j.jinorgbio.2017.02.001

[60] Xiong L, Liu Z, Ouyang G, et al. Autophagy inhibition enhances photocytotoxicity of Photosan-II in human colorectal cancer cells. Oncotarget. 2017;**8**(4):6419-6432. DOI: 10.18632/oncotarget.14117

[61] Yuzhakova DV, Lermontova SA, Grigoryev IS, et al. In vivo multimodal tumor imaging and photodynamic therapy with novel theranostic agents based on the porphyrazine framework-chelated gadolinium (III) cation. Biochimica et Biophysica Acta—General Subjects. 2017;**1861**(12):3120-3130. DOI: 10.1016/j.bbagen.2017.09.004

[62] Rocha LB, Schaberle F, Dąbrowski JM, et al. Intravenous single-dose toxicity of redaporfin-based photodynamic therapy in rodents. International Journal of Molecular Sciences. 2015;**16**(12):29236-29249. DOI: 10.3390/ijms161226162

[63] Sun B, Li W, Liu N. Curative effect of the recent photofrin photodynamic adjuvant treatment on young patients with advanced colorectal cancer. Oncology Letters. 2016;**11**:2071-2074. DOI: 10.3892/ol.2016.4179

[64] Hon EJ, Choi DG, Shim MS. Targeted and effective photodynamic therapy for cancer using functionalized nanomaterials. Acta Pharmaceutica Sinica B. 2016;**6**(4):297-307. DOI: 10.1016/j.apsb.2016.01.007

[65] Lim CK, Heo J, Shin S, et al. Nanophotosensitizers toward advanced photodynamic therapy of cancer. Cancer Letters. 2013;**334**(2):176-187. DOI: 10.1016/j.canlet.2012.09.012

[66] Manikandan M, Kannan K, Manavalan R, et al. Design of nanoparticles for colon target drug delivery—A review. Research Journal of Pharmaceutical, Biological and Chemical Sciences. 2011;**2**(4):128-139

[67] Hamzehzadeh L, Imanparast A, Tajbakhsh A, et al. New approaches to use nanoparticles for treatment of colorectal cancer: A brief review. Nanomedicine Research Journal. 2016;**1**(2):59-68. DOI: 10.7508/nmrj.2016.02.001

[68] Varol M. An alternative treatment modality of diseases using photodynamic therapy with a wide range biological targeting possibility. Research & Reviews: Research Journal of Biology. 2015;**3**:21-25

[69] Sarangi MJ, Pahi S. Colon targeted drug delivery system—An approach for treating colonic ailments. Critical Review. 2015;**2**(3):9-10

[70] Gaware VS, Håkerud M, Juzeniene A, et al. Endosome targeting meso-tetraphenylchlorin-chitosan nanoconjugates for photochemical internalization. Biomacromolecules. 2017;**18**(4):1108-1126. DOI: 10.1021/acs.biomac.6b01670

[71] Pramual S, Assavanig A, Bergkvist M, et al. Development

and characterization of bio-derived polyhydroxyalkanoate nanoparticles as a delivery system for hydrophobic photodynamic therapy agents. Journal of Materials Science. Materials in Medicine. 2016;**27**(2):40. DOI: 10.1007/s10856-015-5655-4

[72] Lee HL, Jeong YL, Kang DH. 5-aminolevulinic acid incorporated nanoparticles of methoxy poly(ethylene glycol)-chitosan copolymer for photodynamic therapy. International Journal of Nanomedicine. 2015;**8**:809-819. DOI: 10.2147/IJN.S39615

[73] Yang SJ, Shieh MJ, Lin FH, et al. Colorectal cancer cell detection by 5-aminolaevulinic acid-loaded chitosan nanoparticles. Cancer Letters. 2009;**273**(2):210-220. DOI: 10.1016/j.canlet.2008.08.014

[74] Yassin AEB, Anwer MK, Mowafy HA, et al. Optimization of 5-flurouracil solid-lipid nanoparticles: A preliminary study to treat colon cancer. International Journal of Medical Sciences. 2010;**7**(6):398-408

[75] Ryu JH, Jeong YI, Kim HY, et al. Enhanced photosensing and photodynamic treatment of colon cancer cells using methoxy poly(ethylene glycol)-conjugated chlorin e6. Journal of Nanoscience and Nanotechnology. 2018;**18**(2):1131-1136. DOI: 10.1166/jnn.2018.14872

[76] Gavrina AI, Shirmanova MV, Aksenova NA, et al. Photodynamic therapy of mouse tumor model using chlorin e6- polyvinyl alcohol complex. Journal of Photochemistry and Photobiology. B. 2018;**178**:614-622. DOI: 10.1016/j.jphotobiol.2017.12.016

[77] Kim DH, Hwang HS, Na K. Photoresponsive micelle-incorporated doxorubicin for chemo-photodynamic therapy to achieve synergistic antitumor effects. Biomacromolecules. 2018;**19**(8):3301-3310. DOI: 10.1021/acs.biomac.8b00607

[78] Anitha A, Deepa N, Chennazhi KP, et al. Combinatorial anticancer effects of curcumin and 5-fluorouracil loaded thiolated chitosan nanoparticles towards colon cancer treatment. Biochimica et Biophysica Acta. 2014;**1840**(9):2730-2743. DOI: 10.1016/j.bbagen.2014.06.004

[79] Kulbacka J, Pucek A, Kotulska M, et al. Electroporation and lipid nanoparticles with cyanine IR-780 and flavonoids as efficient vectors to enhanced drug delivery in colon cancer. Bioelectrochemistry. 2016;**110**:19-31. DOI: 10.1016/j.bioelechem.2016.02.013

[80] Ballestri M, Caruso E, Guerrini A, et al. Core-shell poly-methyl methacrylate nanoparticles covalently functionalized with a non-symmetric porphyrin for anticancer photodynamic therapy. Journal of Photochemistry and Photobiology. B. 2018;**186**:169-177. DOI: 10.1016/j.jphotobiol.2018.07.013

[81] Wong RCH, Chow SYS, Zhao S, et al. pH-Responsive dimeric zinc(II) phthalocyanine in mesoporous silica nanoparticles as an activatable nanophotosensitizing system for photodynamic therapy. ACS Applied Materials & Interfaces. 2017;**9**(28):23487-23496. DOI: 10.1021/acsami.7b06353

[82] Montanha MC, Silva LL, Pangoni FBB, et al. Response surface method optimization of a novel Hypericin formulation in P123 micelles for colorectal cancer and antimicrobial photodynamic therapy. Journal of Photochemistry and Photobiology. B. 2017;**170**:247-255. DOI: 10.1016/j.jphotobiol.2017.04.008

[83] Tamai K, Mizushima T, Wu X, et al. Photodynamic therapy using indocyanine green loaded on super carbonate apatite as minimally invasive

cancer treatment. Molecular Cancer Therapeutics. 2018;**17**(7):1613-1622. DOI: 10.1158/1535-7163.MCT-17-0788

[84] Nagy-Simon T, Potara M, Craciun AM, et al. IR780-dye loaded gold nanoparticles as new near infrared activatable nanotheranostic agents for simultaneous photodynamic and photothermal therapy and intracellular tracking by surface enhanced resonant Raman scattering imaging. Journal of Colloid and Interface Science. 2018;**517**:239-250. DOI: 10.1016/j.jcis.2018.02.007

[85] Wu RW, Chu ES, Huang Z, et al. An *in vitro* investigation of photodynamic efficacy of FosPeg® on human colon cancer cells. Journal of Innovative Optical Health Sciences. 2015;**8**(5):1550027. DOI: 10.1142/S1793545815500273

[86] Wang X, Yuan B, Dong W, et al. Induction of heat-shock protein 70 expression by geranylgeranylacetone shows cytoprotective effects in cardiomyocytes of mice under humid heat stress. PLoS One. 2014;**9**(4):e93536. DOI: 10.1371/journal.pone.0093536

[87] Ogawara K, Shiraishi T, Araki T, et al. Efficient anti-tumor effect of photodynamic treatment with polymeric nanoparticles composed of polyethylene glycol and polylactic acid block copolymer encapsulating hydrophobic porphyrin derivative. European Journal of Pharmaceutical Sciences. 2016;**82**:154-160. DOI: 10.1016/j.ejps.2015.11.016

[88] Viard M, Reichard H, Shapiro BA, et al. Design and biological activity of novel stealth polymeric lipid nanoparticles for enhanced delivery of hydrophobic photodynamic therapy drugs. Nanomedicine. 2018;**14**(7):2295-2305. DOI: 10.1016/j.nano.2018.07.006

[89] Yang X, Xue X, Luo Y, et al. Sub-100 nm, long tumor retention SN-38-loaded photonic micelles for tri-modal cancer therapy. Journal of Controlled Release. 2017;**261**:297-306. DOI: 10.1016/j.jconrel.2017.07.014

[90] Simon V, Devaux C, Darmon A, et al. Pp IX silica nanoparticles demonstrate differential interactions with *in vitro* tumor cell lines and *in vivo* mouse models of human cancers. Photochemistry and Photobiology. 2010;**86**(1):213-222. DOI: 10.1111/j.1751-1097.2009.00620.x

[91] Peng CL, Lai PS, Lin FH, et al. Dual chemotherapy and photodynamic therapy in an HT-29 human colon cancer xenograft model using SN-38-loaded chlorin-core star block copolymer micelles. Biomaterials. 2009;**30**(21):3614-3625. DOI: 10.1016/j.biomaterials.2009.03.048

[92] Bakhshizadeh M, Moshirian T, Esmaily H, et al. Sonophotodynamic therapy mediated by liposomal zinc phthalocyanine in a colon carcinoma tumor model: Role of irradiating arrangement. Iranian Journal of Basic Medical Sciences. 2017;**20**(10):1088-1092. DOI: 10.22038/IJBMS.2017.9410

[93] Yurt F, Ince M, Colak SG, et al. Investigation of *in vitro* PDT activities of zinc phthalocyanine immobilised TiO2 nanoparticles. International Journal of Pharmaceutics. 2017;**524**(1-2):467-474. DOI: 10.1016/j.ijpharm.2017.03.050

[94] Fang J, Liao L, Yin H, et al. Photodynamic therapy and imaging based on tumor-targeted nanoprobe, polymer-conjugated zinc protoporphyrin. Future Science OA. 2015;**1**(3):FSO4. DOI: 10.4155/fso.15.2

[95] Chiarante N, García Vior MC, Awruch J, et al. Phototoxic action of a zinc(II) phthalocyanine encapsulated into poloxamine polymeric micelles in 2D and 3D colon carcinoma cell cultures. Journal of Photochemistry and

Photobiology. B. 2017;**170**:140-151. DOI: 10.1016/j.jphotobiol.2017.04.009

[96] Alexis F, Pridgen EM, Langer R, et al. Nanoparticle technologies for cancer therapy. Handbook of Experimental Pharmacology. 2010;**197**:55-86. DOI: 10.1007/978-3-642-00477-3_2

[97] Atena M, Mohammad Reza A, Mehran G. A review on the biology of cancer stem cells. Stem Cell Discovery. 2014;**4**:83-89. DOI: 10.4236/scd.2014.44009

[98] Chen K, Huang YH, Chen JL. Understanding and targeting cancer stem cells: Therapeutic implications and challenges. Acta Pharmacologica Sinica. 2013;**34**(6):732-740. DOI: 10.1038/aps.2013.27

[99] Yang L, He J, Wen Y, et al. Nanoscale photodynamic agents for colorectal cancer treatment: A review. Journal of Biomedical Nanotechnology. 2016;**12**(7):1348-1373

[100] Ferreira CS, Cheung MC, Missailidis S, et al. Phototoxic aptamers selectively enter and kill epithelial cancer cells. Nucleic Acids Research. 2009;**37**(3):866-876. DOI: 10.1093/nar/gkn967

[101] Bhatti M, Yahioglu G, Milgrom LR, et al. Targeted photodynamic therapy with multiply-loaded recombinant antibody fragments. International Journal of Cancer. 2008;**122**(5):1155-1163. DOI: 10.1002/ijc.23206

[102] Isaac-Lam MF, Hammonds DM. Biotinylated chlorin and its zinc and indium complexes: Synthesis and *In vitro* biological evaluation for photodynamic therapy. Pharmaceuticals (Basel). 2017;**10**(2):E41, 10.3390/ph10020041

[103] Yang S, Gao H. Nanoparticles for modulating tumor microenvironment to improve drug delivery and tumor therapy. Pharmacological Research. 2017;**126**:97-108. DOI: 10.1016/j.phrs.2017.05.004

[104] Gao S, Wang J, Tian R, et al. Construction and evaluation of a targeted hyaluronic acid nanoparticle/photosensitizer complex for cancer photodynamic therapy. ACS Applied Materials & Interfaces. 2017;**9**(38):32509-32519. DOI: 10.1021/acsami.7b09331

[105] Tanaka M, Kataoka H, Yano S, et al. Immunogenic cell death due to a new photodynamic therapy (PDT) with glycoconjugated chlorin (G-chlorin). Oncotarget. 2016;**7**(30):47242-47251. DOI: 10.18632/oncotarget.9725

[106] Halaburková A, Jendželovský R, Koval' J, et al. Histone deacetylase inhibitors potentiate photodynamic therapy in colon cancer cells marked by chromatin-mediated epigenetic regulation of CDKN1A. Clinical Epigenetics. 2017;**9**:62. DOI: 10.1186/s13148-017-0359-x

[107] Wang K, Zhang Y, Wang J, et al. Self-assembled IR780-loaded transferrin nanoparticles as an imaging, targeting and PDT/PTT agent for cancer therapy. Scientific Reports. 2016;**6**:27421. DOI: 10.1038/srep27421

[108] Del Governatore M, Hamblin MR, Piccinini EE, et al. Targeted photodestruction of human colon cancer cells using charged Dougherty chlorine6immunoconjugates. British Journal of Cancer. 2000;**82**(1):56-64. DOI: 10.1054/bjoc.1999.0877

[109] Peng CL, Lin HC, Chiang WL, et al. Anti-angiogenic treatment (Bevacizumab) improves the responsiveness of photodynamic therapy in colorectal cancer. Photodiagnosis and Photodynamic Therapy. 2018;**23**:111-118. DOI: 10.1016/j.pdpdt.2018.06.008

[110] Azhdarzadeh M, Atyabi F, Saei AA, et al. Theranostic MUC-1 aptamer targeted gold coated superparamagnetic iron oxide nanoparticles for magnetic resonance imaging and photothermal therapy of colon cancer. Colloids and Surfaces. B, Biointerfaces. 2016;**143**:224-232. DOI: 10.1016/j.colsurfb.2016.02.058

[111] Subudhi MB, Jain A, Jain A, et al. Eudragit S100 coated citrus pectin nanoparticles for colon targeting of 5-fluorouracil. Materials. 2015;**8**(3):832-849. DOI: 10.3390/ma8030832

[112] Park H, Ko SH, Lee JM, et al. Troglitazone enhances the apoptotic response of DLD-1 colon cancer cells to photodynamic therapy. Yonsei Medical Journal. 2016;**57**(6):1494-1499. DOI: 10.3349/ymj.2016.57.6.1494

[113] Obaid G, Chambrier I, Cook MJ, et al. Cancer targeting with biomolecules: A comparative study of photodynamic therapy efficacy using antibody or lectin conjugated phthalocyanine-PEG gold nanoparticles. Photochemical & Photobiological Sciences. 2015;**14**(4):737-747. DOI: 10.1039/c4pp00312h

Section 5

Multidisciplinary Approach for Prognostic Prediction

Chapter 5

Immunoscore and Microbiome in Colorectal Cancer: What's New?

Filipa Macedo, Nuno Bonito, Adhemar Longatto-Filho and Sandra F. Martins

Abstract

Colorectal cancer (CRC) is the third most commonly diagnosed malignancy and the fourth leading cause of cancer death in the world, accounting for about 1.4 million new cases and almost 700,000 deaths in 2012. The clinical outcome and the tumor progression are now considered the result of a balance between the invasiveness of the tumor and the immune response of the patient against the tumor. The immune system has the ability to control and shape cancer through a mechanism called immunoediting, which include elimination, equilibrium, and escape. The consensus Immunoscore is a scoring system that outlines the density of CD3+ and CD8+ T-cell effectors existent in the tumor and its invasive margin. The pre-existing intra-tumoral immunity could be enhanced and activated by immunotherapy. Immunoscore could be a good prognostic marker, by identifying patients at high risk of tumor recurrence and stratifying patients who could benefit from adjuvant therapies. Human surfaces and cavities are populated by numerous microbial communities, and they play an indispensable role in human health, as they interact with the immune system. The authors made a literature revision concerning the role of Immunoscore and microbiome in colorectal cancer.

Keywords: colorectal cancer, Immunoscore, microbiome, diet, CD3+ T cell, CD8+ T cell

1. Colorectal cancer facts

Colorectal cancer (CRC) is the third most commonly diagnosed malignancy and the fourth leading cause of cancer death in the world, accounting for about 1.4 million new cases and almost 700,000 deaths in 2012 [1]. In Portugal, the incidence of CRC is 42.80 new cases for 100,000 habitants with a mortality rate of 26.6 [2]. The distribution of CRC burden varies widely around the world, with more than two-thirds of all cases and about 60% of all deaths occurring in developed countries. The global burden of CRC is expected to increase by 60% to more than 2.2 million new cases and 1.1 million cancer deaths by 2030 [1]. The lifetime risk of developing colorectal cancer is about 6%, which increased fourfold if there is a family history of CRC.

The multistep models of CRC tumorigenesis postulate an adenoma-carcinoma sequence as the main pathway to develop a cancer. It tells us that CRC arises from a benign precursor polyp that became dysplastic and invasive due to accumulative mutations [3].

 IntechOpen

There are several risk factors for CRC: inherited predisposition (the involvement of at least one first-degree relative doubles the risk, and the risk is even higher if the affected case was prior to the age of 60), obesity, total caloric intake, red meat, sedentary lifestyle and physical inactivity, alcohol consumption, and prolonged cigarette smoking. A low incidence of CRC is associated with high-fiber diet (it dilutes fecal carcinogens, decreases colon transit time, and generates a favorable luminal environment), fruits and vegetables, aspirin, and nonsteroidal anti-inflammatory drugs [4].

An anatomic shift is being observed once the incidence of right-sided or proximal cancer is rising. This shift is due to increased longevity, a response to luminal carcinogens and genetic defects like defects in mismatch repair genes with resulting microsatellite instability (MSI) in proximal colon cancers and chromosomal instability pathway (CIN) in left-sided colon cancer.

Since 2015, there are five consensus molecular subtypes (CMS) of CRC [5]. The CMS1 is the MSI-immune and accounts for 14% of the cancers. This subtype is characterized by proximal colon locations, high BRAF V600E mutation rate, hypermethylation of CpG islands which causes loss of tumor suppressor function, an association with an impaired DNA mismatch repair (MMR) system, an infiltration of immunogenic lymphocytes in the microenvironment, and MSI. MSI cancers are also considered "hypermutated" with approximately 47 mutations per 106 bases, compared to microsatellite stable (MSS or CMS2) tumors which average 2.8/106 bases. The clinical implications of this subtype are that early stage MSI tumors (most CMS1 cancers) have better prognosis than MSS cancers. Stage II cancers with MSI have a low recurrence rate and thus are generally not considered for adjuvant chemotherapy. Patients with stage III MSI tumors do not benefit from fluorouracil monotherapy but are responsive to combination fluorouracil, leucovorin, and oxaliplatin (FOLFOX) adjuvant chemotherapy. CMS1 tumors have a favorable outcome when detected before disease dissemination. In part, the good prognosis may be linked to the presence of specific T-cell populations: CD8+ cytotoxic T lymphocytes, CD4+ activated type 1 T helper cells (Th1), and natural killer cells. However, CMS1 tumors were associated with worse survival after relapse [5, 6]. The CMS2 is the canonical subtype and accounts for 37% of the cancers. This subtype is characterized by a low mutation rate. Five-year overall survival for all stages of CMS2 is the highest, and it has the highest survival rate after relapse. Additionally, CMS2 cancers were more commonly left-sided lesions (59%) [5, 6]. The CMS3 is the metabolic subtype and accounts for 13% of the cancers. This subtype is characterized by RAS mutations (68% of the cancers) which predict poor response to epidermal growth factor receptor (EGFR) monoclonal antibodies (e.g., cetuximab) [5, 6]. The CMS4 is the mesenchymal subtype and accounts for 23% of the cancers. This subtype is characterized by very high pro-inflammatory microenvironment. Additionally, they exhibit extremely low levels of hypermutation and are MSS status. CMS4 cancers, often diagnosed at advanced stages, have a poor prognosis with the worst 5-year overall survival (62%) and relapse-free survival (60%) of any molecular subtype. Although standard adjuvant therapy (FOLFOX) for stage III is recommended, CMS4 cancers show no benefit from systemic adjuvant treatments.

For metastatic disease, CMS4 cancers are resistant to anti-EGFR therapy, independent of RAS mutation status. Anti-angiogenesis therapies such as bevacizumab are standard additions for stage IV disease [5, 6]. Finally, the last subtype is the mixed features and accounts for 13% of the cancers [5, 6].

There are four stages of colon cancer considering their size, number of lymph nodes, and distant metastasis (TNM). Stage 1 comprehends the T1 and T2 tumors (extension to submucosa and muscularis propria), and the treatment is only chirurgical. Stage 2 englobes the T3 and T4 tumors (subserosa, invasion of visceral peritoneum and organs), and the treatment depends if the patient is considered of low or high risk. The low-risk patients only do surgery; the high-risk patients have 1 of the following criteria: less than 12 lymph nodes resected; low differentiated tumor; vascular, lymphatic, or perineural invasion; perforation or intestinal obstruction; T4 tumor; and MSS status. The high-risk stage II and stage III (with lymph nodes positive for disease) patients are submitted to adjuvant chemotherapy after surgery with fluoropirimidine and oxaliplatin. Stage IV cancer is a metastatic disease, which could be resected if feasible or controlled with chemotherapy.

2. What is an Immunoscore?

The clinical outcome and the tumor progression are now considered the result of a balance between the invasiveness of the tumor and the immune response of the patient against the tumor. The immune system has the ability to control and shape cancer through a mechanism called immunoediting, which include elimination, equilibrium, and escape [7].

It was already shown that the strength of the in situ adaptive immune reaction is strongly correlated with time to recurrence and overall survival of CRC [8]. This in situ immune cell infiltration in cancer, called high density of tumor-infiltrating lymphocytes (TIL), is associated with a favorable prognostic effect [8]. Once cancer becomes clinically detectable, the adaptive immune response plays a critical role in preventing tumor recurrence, metastization, and clinical outcome. A protective response is maintained by the ability of memory T cells to recall previously encountered antigens [9]. Concerning to regulatory T cells (Tregs), Sinicrope et al. showed an association between a low CD3+/FoxP3+ cell ratio and shorter survival [10], but Salama et al. showed the opposite, a high Treg density in the tumor was associated with improved survival [11]. Regarding TH17 and TH1 immune response, TH17 is associated with poor prognosis [12], and TH1 is associated with prolonged disease-free survival [13].

The consensus Immunoscore is a scoring system that outlines the density of CD3+ and CD8+ T-cell effectors existent in the tumor and its invasive margin. The pre-existing intra-tumoral immunity could be enhanced and activated by immunotherapy. Immunoscore could be a good prognostic marker, by identifying patients at high risk of tumor recurrence and stratifying patients who could benefit from adjuvant therapies [14]. This score is based in the numeration of two lymphocyte populations (CD3/CD45RO, CD3/CD8 or CD8/CD45RO), in density (Cells/mm2) and the location (in the core of the tumor or in the invasive margin) [15]. The score ranges from Immunoscore 0 (I0) when low densities of both cell types are found in both regions to Immunoscore 4 (I4) when high densities are found in both regions.

3. Clinical applications of Immunoscore

Immunoscore has been tested to be a prognostic marker that surpasses the TNM staging. Pages et al. concluded that patients with high Immunoscore had the lowest risk of recurrence and longest survival. In his study, only 5% of the patients with high Immunoscore had a recurrence at 3 years, 87% of the patients reached the overall survival at 3 years, and 82% of the patients reached 5-year overall survival [14].

There is a possible association between MSI status and immune cell infiltrates. MSI-high tumors have intraepithelial T cells due to expression of neo-antigens on the cell surface, and this could be the reason why this kind of tumors had better prognosis [15].

Comparing to the American Joint Committee on Cancer/Union for International Cancer Control (AJCC/UICC) TNM classification system, the Immunoscore classification seems to be superior as prognostic tool. For all patients with CRC stages I/II/III, multivariate Cox analysis revealed that the immune criteria remained highly associated with prognosis [16]. Wirta et al. concluded that a lower Immunoscore was associated with increasing AJCC/UICC stage, as well as with increasing T stage, presence of lymph node, distant metastasis, and perineural or lymphovascular invasion [17].

One day the classification of cancer will have a new component, TNM-I (immune).

Additionally, Immunoscore can predict the response to treatment and could be a biomarker that helps clinicians to decide what patients must have chemotherapy. Morris et al. concluded that high TIL is predictive of response to chemotherapy with 5-fluorouracil [18], and Viaud et al. revealed that cyclophosphamide induces a TH17 and TH1 antitumor response, making the tumors resistant to this chemotherapy [19].

4. What is a microbiome?

Human surfaces and cavities are populated by numerous microbial communities, like bacteria or fungi, which form a complex interactive network between themselves and the host. The gastrointestinal microbiota is estimated to contain over 1000 different phylotypes with a microbial gene catalog of 3.3 million genes [20], but it can be divided into four main categories: *Firmicutes*, *Bacteroides*, *Actinobacteria*, and *Proteobacteria* [21]. These agents play an indispensable role in human health, as they interact with the immune system, maintain epithelial homeostasis, metabolize indigestible polysaccharides, modulate the intestinal motility, regulate the luminal pH, and exclude potential pathogens from the human gut [22]. The disruption of intestinal microbial equilibrium has the capacity to alter the homeostatic network, thereby eliciting deleterious host responses as observed in inflammatory bowel disease and CRC. The dysbiosis refers to perturbations in microbial populations [23].

Wong et al. proved that intestinal microbiota has an important role in CRC carcinogenesis. Mice fed with stool from patients with CRC had a higher rate of high-grade dysplasia than the mice fed with stool from healthy controls, suggesting that human commensals may not be tumorigenic [24]. Bacteria may contribute to CRC in several ways: they can break the mucus layer and adhere to intestinal mucosa and deliver virulent proteins and molecules that will initiate oncogenic signaling in epithelial cells. As so, they can induce DNA damage leading to tumor initiation. On the other hand, bacteria can trigger procarcinogenic signaling and inflammatory microenvironment, such as IL-17 production or excessive Wnt or Stat3 signaling [25].

Some studies have identified several bacteria that can promote carcinogenesis by different mechanisms: *Escherichia coli* can cause direct DNA damage such as crosslinks and double-strand breaks due to the colibactin toxin produced by it [26], *Fusobacterium nucleatum* can produce FadA adhesin to modulate E-cadherin/beta-catenin signaling [27], *Peptostreptococcus anaerobius* can induce cell proliferation through toll-like receptor 2 and toll-like receptor 4 pathways [28], *Bacteroides fragilis* produces a toxin that activates Wnt and NF-kB pathways which induce a pro-inflammatory state [29], and *Streptococcus gallolyticus* induces tumor growth through enhancement of inflammatory signals including cyclooxygenase-2 [30].

Xu et al. compared normal tissue with adenomas and adenocarcinomas and concluded that the microorganisms are different between the three entities. In the cancer group, 20 biomarkers were identified: *Bulleidia*, *Catonella*, *Clostridium*, *Dialister*, *Granulicatella*, *Lactobacillus*, *Mogibacterium*, *Oscillospira*, *Parvimonas*, *Peptostreptococcus*, *Streptococcus*, *Odoribacter*, *Paraprevotella*, *Porphyromonas*, *Prevotella*, *Fusobacterium*, *Leptotrichia*, *Campylobacter*, *Desulfovibrio*, and *Treponema* [31].

Even in the same individual, there are differences between normal and disease tissue sites. One study compared cancerous tissue with matched healthy tissue, and the microbial diversity was significantly lower in tumor tissue, suggesting a more selective microenvironment in proximity to diseased tissue [32].

5. Clinical applications of microbiome analysis

Some studies stablish a relationship between the microbiota and the cancer therapy efficacy. Iida et al. showed that microbiota leads to enzyme expression required for optimal chemotherapy activity with oxaliplatin [18]. Guthrie et al. demonstrated that inhibition of microbial ß-glucuronidase increases the adverse effects of irinotecan in some patients [33]. Concerning immunotherapy, a great number of bacteria were observed having great clinical response to immune-checkpoint therapy (by activating CTLA-4 and PD1 expression or promoting T-cell proliferation) [34].

Nevertheless, the main application nowadays is the fecal microbiota transplantation. This procedure consists in the administration of fecal bacteria from a healthy donor (without cancer, an autoimmune or metabolic disease) to a recipient by enema, colonoscopy, or enteric tube. The main objective is to alter the recipient's microbiota composition, and it is performed in a variety of diseases like *Clostridium difficile* infection, irritable bowel syndrome, inflammatory bowel diseases, obesity, multiple sclerosis, and type 2 diabetes mellitus [35]. Unfortunately, the lack of evidence and clinical trials bounds their use in clinical practice of oncologic patients.

Another potential application is through oral probiotics. Probiotics are supplements with live bacteria that promote gut health. Some experimental models presented a reduction rate of colorectal cancer development with their consumption [36].

6. Diet

Some dietary compounds may reach the colon by several reasons: they could be too large to be absorbed in the small intestine, they could escape the deglycosylation and absorption in the small intestine, and they could not be accessible to the host due to the mixture of food. The dietary compounds that are absorbed in the small intestine could reach the colon by enterohepatic circulation [37]. Dietary bioactives can modify the carcinogenic process in several ways: by a direct or microbe-independent pathway and by an indirect or microbe-dependent pathway that include modifications in the substrates that alter the colonic microbiota or their metabolites [38]. The dietary fiber goes through the small intestine into the cecum and proximal colon where they are metabolized by the colonic microbiota and short-chain fatty acids are produced [39]. The most abundant short-chain fatty acids in the colon are acetate, propionate, and butyrate, and their concentrations typically decrease from the proximal to the distal colon [40]. The advantages from consuming fibers are the dilution of carcinogens and potential tumor promoters in the intestinal lumen [41] and the fast passage of the digesta through the colon which minimize the exposition to toxic products and increase the levels of short-chain fatty acids in the distal colon [42].

Butyrate is the preferred substrate of colonocytes [43]. This compost was incredibly studied due to its capacity to reduce oxidative stress, diminish inflammation and carcinogenesis, and support colonic barrier function [44].

The diet can shape the colonic microbiota and their function, and, on the other hand, the microbiota influences the health of the intestine. This way the host is protected from colon cancer and other inflammatory diseases.

7. Conclusions

CRC is the third most commonly diagnosed malignancy and the fourth leading cause of cancer death in the world. There are five CMS of CRC: the MSI-immune, the canonical subtype, the metabolic subtype, and the last subtype with mixed features. The strength of the in situ adaptive immune reaction is strongly correlated with time to recurrence and overall survival of CRC which leads us to think that the immune system plays an important role in CRC development. The consensus Immunoscore is a scoring system that outlines the density of CD3+ and CD8+ T-cell effectors existent in the tumor and its invasive margin, and the authors believe that this score could be a good prognostic marker. On the other hand, the dysbiosis could be combined with Immunoscore to increase the power of the biomarker. Studies about this interaction are needed. The role of microbiota in colorectal cancer is complex: its disturbance is the cause of tumorigenesis, or the outcome of tumor development is still uncertain.

Conflict of interest

The authors have no conflict of interest.

DOI: http://dx.doi.org/10.5772/intechopen.86605

Author details

Filipa Macedo[1], Nuno Bonito[1], Adhemar Longatto-Filho[2,3,4,5]
and Sandra F. Martins[2,3,6]*

1 Portuguese Oncology Institute, Coimbra, Portugal

2 Life and Health Science Research Institute (ICVS), School of Medicine, University of Minho, Braga, Portugal

3 ICVS/3B's-PT Government Associate Laboratory, Braga/Guimarães, Braga, Portugal

4 Molecular Oncology Research Center, Barretos, São Paulo, Brazil

5 Laboratory of Medical Investigation (LIM) 14, Faculty of Medicine, University of Sao Paulo, Brazil

6 Surgery Department, Coloproctology Unit, Braga Hospital, Braga, Portugal

*Address all correspondence to: sandramartins@med.uminho.pt

References

[1] Ferlay J, Soerjomataram I, Ervik M, et al. GLOBOCAN 2012 v1.0, Cancer Incidence and Mortality Worldwide: IARC Cancer Base No. 11. Lyon, France: International Agency for Research on Cancer; 2013

[2] Doenças Oncológicas em números—2013. Direcção geral da saúde. ISSN: 2183-0746

[3] Leslie A, Carey F, Pratt N, Steele R. The colorectal adenoma-carcinoma sequence. The British Journal of Surgery. 2002;**89**(7):845-860

[4] DeVita, Hellman, and Rosenberg's Cancer: Principles & Practice of Oncology. 10th ed. Wolters Kluwer; chapter 56 - Molecular Biology of Colorectal Cancer. pp. 757-767

[5] Müller M, Ibrahim A, Arends M. Molecular pathological classification of colorectal cancer. Virchows Archiv. 2016;**469**:125-134

[6] Thanki K, Nicholls M, Gajjar A, Senagore A, Qiu S, Szabo C, et al. Consensus molecular subtypes of colorectal cancer and their clinical implications. International Biological and Biomedical Journal. 2017;**3**(3):105-111

[7] Dunn G, Old L, Schreiber R. The three Es of cancer immunoediting. Annual Review of Immunology. 2004;**22**:329-360

[8] Galon J, Costes A, Sanchez-Cabo F, et al. Type, density, and location of immune cells within human colorectal tumours predict clinical outcome. Science. 2006;**313**:1960-1964

[9] Sallusto F, Geginat J, Lanzavecchia A. Central memory and effector memory T cell subsets: Function, generation, and maintenance. Annual Review of Immunology. 2004;**22**:745-763

[10] Sinicrope F, Rego R, Ansell S, Knutson K, Foster N, Sargent D. Intraepithelial effector (CD3+)/regulatory (FoxP3+) T-cell ratio predicts a clinical outcome of human colon carcinoma. Gastroenterology. 2009;**137**:1270-1279

[11] Salama P, Phillips M, Grieu F, Morris M, Zeps N, Joseph D, et al. Tumor-infiltrating FOXP3+ T regulatory cells show strong prognostic significance in colorectal cancer. Journal of Clinical Oncology. 2009;**27**:186-192

[12] Wu S, Rhee K, Albesiano E, Rabizadeh S, Wu X, et al. A human colonic commensal promotes colon tumorigenesis via activation of T helper type 17 T cell responses. Nature Medicine. 2009;**15**:1016-1022

[13] Tosolini M, Kirilovsky A, Mlecnik B, Fredriksen T, Mauger S, Bindea G, et al. Clinical impact of different classes of infiltrating T cytotoxic and helper cells (Th1, th2, treg, th17) in patients with colorectal cancer. Cancer Research. 2011;**71**:1263-1271

[14] Pagès F, Mlecnik B, Marliot F, Bindea G, Ou F, et al. International validation of the consensus Immunoscore for the classification of colon cancer: A prognostic and accuracy study. Lancet. 2018;**391**(10135):2128-2139

[15] Galon J, Mlecnik B, Bindea G, Angell H, Berger A, et al. Towards the introduction of the 'Immunoscore' in the classification of malignant tumours. The Journal of Pathology. 2014;**232**(2):199-209

[16] Mlecnik B, Tosolini M, Kirilovsky A, et al. Histopathologic-based prognostic factors of colorectal cancers are associated with the state of the local immune reaction. Journal of Clinical Oncology. 2011;**29**:610-618

[17] Wirta E, Seppala T, Friman M, Vayrynen J, Ahtiainen M, et al. Immunoscore in mismatch repair-proficient and -deficient colon cancer. Journal of Pathology: Clinical Research. 2017;**3**:203-213

[18] Morris M, Platell C, Iacopetta B. Tumor-infiltrating lymphocytes and perforation in colon cancer predict positive response to 5-fluorouracil chemotherapy. Clinical Cancer Research. 2008;**14**:1413-1417

[19] Viaud S, Saccheri F, Mignot G, Yamazaki T, Daillère R, Hannani D, et al. The intestinal microbiota modulates the anticancer immune effects of cyclophosphamide. Science. 2013;**342**:971-976

[20] Lozupone C, Stombaugh J, Gordon J, Jansson J, Knight R. Diversity, stability and resilience of the human gut microbiota. Nature. 2012;**489**:220-230

[21] Qin J, Li R, Raes J, et al. A human gut microbial gene catalogue established by metagenomic sequencing. Nature. 2010;**464**:59-65

[22] Gill S, Pop M, Deboy R, et al. Metagenomic analysis of the human distal gut microbiome. Science. 2006;**312**:1355-1359

[23] Sobhani I, Tap J, Roudot-Thoraval F, Roperch J, Letulle S, Langella P, et al. Microbial dysbiosis in colorectal cancer (CRC) patients. PLoS One. 2011;**6**:e16393

[24] Wong S, Zhao L, Zhang X, Nakatsu G, Han J, Xu W, et al. Gavage of fecal samples from patients with colorectal cancer promotes intestinal carcinogenesis in germ-free and conventional mice. Gastroenterology. 2017;**153**(6):1621-1633.e6

[25] McAllister F, Housseau F, Sears C. Microbiota and immune responses in colon cancer: More to learn. Cancer Journal. 2014;**20**(3):232-236

[26] Cuevas-Ramos G, Petit C, Marcq I, et al. Escherichia coli induces DNA damage in vivo and triggers genomic instability in mammalian cells. Proceedings of the National Academy of Sciences of the United States of America. 2010;**107**:11537-11542

[27] Rubinstein M, Wang X, Liu W, et al. Fusobacterium nucleatum promotes colorectal carcinogenesis by modulating E-cadherin/beta-catenin signaling via its FadA adhesin. Cell Host & Microbe. 2013;**14**:195-206

[28] Tsoi H, Chu E, Zhang X, et al. Peptostreptococcus anaerobius induces intracellular cholesterol biosynthesis in colon cells to induce proliferation and causes dysplasia in mice. Gastroenterology. 2017;**152**:1419-1433.e5

[29] Goodwin A, Shields C, Wu S, Huso D, Wu X, Murray- Stewart T, et al. Polyamine catabolism contributes to enterotoxigenic Bacteroides fragilis-induced colon tumorigenesis. Proceedings of the National Academy of Sciences of the United States of America. 2011;**108**:15354-15359

[30] Abdulamir A, Hafidh R, Bakar F. Molecular detection, quantification, and isolation of Streptococcus gallolyticus bacteria colonizing Colorectal tumors: Inflammation-driven potential of carcinogenesis via IL-1, COX-2, and IL-8. Molecular Cancer. 2010;**9**:249

[31] Xu K, Jiang B. Analysis of mucosa-associated microbiota in colorectal cancer. Medical Science Monitor. 2017;**23**:4422-4430

[32] Chen W, Liu F, Ling Z, Tong X, Xiang C. Human intestinal lumen and mucosa-associated microbiota in patients with colorectal cancer. PLoS One. 2012;7:e39743

[33] Guthrie L, Gupta S, Daily J, Kelly L. Human microbiome signatures of differential colorectal cancer drug metabolism. npj Biofilms and Microbiomes. 2017;**3**:27

[34] Matson V, Fessler J, Bao R, Chongsuwat T, Zha Y, Alegre ML, et al. The commensal microbiome is associated with anti-PD-1 efficacy in metastatic melanoma patients. Science. 2018;**359**(6371):104-108

[35] Smits L, Bouter K, de Vos W, Borody T, Nieuwdorp M. Therapeutic potential of fecal microbiota transplantation. Gastroenterology. 2013;**145**(5):946-953

[36] Del Carmen S, de Moreno de LeBlanc A, Levit R, Azevedo V, Langella P, Bermúdez-Humarán L, et al. Anti-cancer effect of lactic acid bacteria expressing antioxidant enzymes or IL-10 in a colorectal cancer mouse model. International Immunopharmacology. 2017;**42**:122-129

[37] Iida N, Dzutsev A, Stewart C, Smith L, Bouladoux N, Weingarten R, et al. Commensal bacteria control cancer response to therapy by modulating the tumor microenvironment. Science. 2013;**342**:967-970

[38] Aura AM. Microbial metabolism of dietary phenolic compounds in the colon. Phytochemistry Reviews. 2008;**7**:407-429

[39] Irrazábal T, Belcheva A, Girardin SE, Martin A, Philpott DJ. The multifaceted role of the intestinal microbiota in colon cancer. Molecular Cell. 2014;**54**:309-320

[40] Turner N, Lupton J. Dietary fiber. Advances in Nutrition. 2011;**2**:151-152

[41] Hamer H, Jonkers D, Venema K, Vanhoutvin S, Troost F, Brummer R. The role of butyrate on colonic function. Alimentary Pharmacology & Therapeutics. 2008;**27**:104-119

[42] Gazzaniga J, Lupton J. Dilution effect of dietary fiber sources: An in vivo study in the rat. Nutrition Research. 1987;**7**:1261-1268

[43] Lewis S, Heaton K. Increasing butyrate concentration in the distal colon by accelerating intestinal transit. Gut. 1997;**41**:245-251

[44] Donohoe D, Curry K, Bultman S. Microbial oncotarget: Bacterial-produced butyrate, chemoprevention and Warburg effect. Oncotarget. 2013;**4**:182-183

Section 6

Understanding Therapeutics for Advanced Colorectal Cancer

Chapter 6

Further Therapeutic Options in Heavily Pretreated Colorectal Cancer Patients

Aneta L. Zygulska

Abstract

In this paper, currently available systemic treatment options (regorafenib, trifluridine/tipiracil, re-challenge chemotherapy, mitomycin C plus capecitabine) for pretreated patients with metastatic colorectal cancer are discussed and compared in terms of their efficacy and safety profiles. Treatment of these patients has remained a challenge for oncologists. The evidence from clinical trials is encouraging. Knowledge of response biomarkers and/or prognostic factors may be helpful in the identification of patients who could benefit most from the treatment. Adequate medication compliance can be achieved due to awareness of toxicity risk among both physicians and cancer patients and appropriate prevention and management of adverse events.

Keywords: metastatic colorectal cancer, regorafenib, trifluridine/tipiracil, re-challenge chemotherapy, mitomycin C plus capecitabine

1. Introduction

To this date, management of heavily pretreated patients with metastatic colorectal cancer, who present with good performance status and adequate organ function reserve, constituted a challenge for oncologists. However, two anticancer therapies dedicated for this specific group of patients became available nowadays. One of them is regorafenib, an oral inhibitor of protein kinases associated with angiogenesis. Another one is trifluridine/tipiracil (TAS-102), an orally administered combination of a thymidine-based nucleic acid analog, and tipiracil hydrochloride, a thymidine phosphorylase inhibitor. Treatment with both anticancer agents contributed to a significant improvement of overall survival (OS) and progression-free survival (PFS) in randomized III phase studies of Caucasian (CORRECT and TERRA) and Asian patients (CONCUR and RECOURSE). Recently, clinical benefits associated with administration of both drugs and good tolerability thereof were also confirmed in an observational study, REGOTAS. The aim of currently ongoing trials is to evaluate the efficacy and safety of regorafenib and TAS-102 combined with other anticancer drugs in metastatic colorectal cancer patients. While preliminary results of some of those studies seem promising, more evidence is needed to formulate any clinically relevant conclusions.

Another treatment option in metastatic colorectal cancer is re-induction of previously used chemotherapy with oxaliplatin- or irinotecan-based regimens.

Importantly, the time elapsed since completion of the primary treatment to the re-induction should not be shorter than 9 months. Finally, patients with metastatic colorectal cancer can receive chemotherapy with mitomycin C plus capecitabine. This generally neglected treatment option seems particularly reasonable in the case of countries in which regorafenib and trifluridine/tipiracil have been registered but are not reimbursed.

The aim of this review paper is to discuss the therapeutic options that could be used in metastatic colorectal cancer patients after three or more lines of systemic therapy.

2. Regorafenib

Regorafenib (BAY 73-4506) is a low-molecular-weight diphenylurea multikinase inhibitor of VEGFR1-3, c-KIT, TIE-2, PDGFR-β, FGFR-1, RET, RAF-1, BRAF, and p38 MAP kinase for oral administration. This agent has been registered for patients with pretreated metastatic colorectal cancers and refractory gastrointestinal stromal tumors (GIST) [1, 2]. Regorafenib is administered at 160 mg daily (q.d.) for 3 weeks of each 4-week cycle (3 week *on*, 1 week *off*), until disease progression or drug intolerance, whichever first.

2.1 Trials

In a registration phase III trial, CORRECT (regorafenib monotherapy for previously treated metastatic colorectal cancer), 760 patients were randomized in a 2:1 ratio to receive regorafenib or placebo. The majority of patients were Caucasians (the study included only 111 Asians). Median OS turned out to be significantly longer in the regorafenib group than in the placebo group (6.4 vs. 5.0 months) [3]. In another randomized double-blind phase III trial, CONCUR, 204 patients with metastatic colorectal cancer after at least two lines of systemic therapy were randomized in a 2:1 ratio to receive regorafenib or placebo. All patients were Asians. Median OS in the regorafenib arm and placebo arm was 8.8 and 6.3 months, respectively. The results of this trial confirmed previous observations about the regorafenib efficacy. Toxicity profiles of regorafenib in both studies mentioned above were essentially similar [4]. However, these promising findings were not confirmed in another trial, PREVIUM, including patients with KRAS- or BRAF-positive metastatic colorectal cancer treated previously with FOLFOXIRI plus bevacizumab; median OS and median PFS in this group were 3.3 and 2.2 months, respectively [5].

2.2 Predictive markers

According to Komori et al., colorectal cancer patients who showed early decrease in carbohydrate antigen 19-9 (Ca19-9) levels had significantly longer PFS after regorafenib than individuals in whom this marker remained elevated (3.7 vs. 2.0 months). Multivariate analysis confirmed that early decrease in Ca19-9 level was a significant independent predictor of better response to regorafenib [6].

The authors of the CORRECT study analyzed an association between mutational status of the tumor and survival. The study demonstrated that the presence of KRAS-wild type and PIK3CA-wild type in primary tumor was a biomarker of PFS benefit [7]. In another study, conducted by Ma et al., the lack of EGFR expression turned out to be associated with longer PFS and OS (14 vs. 2.5 months and 19.7 vs. 9.6 months, respectively). While the presence of KRAS-wild type correlated with longer OS, no significant association was found between this biomarker and PFS [8]. Furthermore, multivariate analysis documented prognostic value of tumor's location in the right or left side of the abdominal cavity, with better prognosis observed in the case of the left-sided malignancies [8].

RECIST 1.1 is an established instrument to assess a response to anticancer treatment based on radiologically determined cumulative diameter of target lesions. Cavitation of lung metastases assessed on CT scans at the baseline and at 8 weeks of regorafenib therapy seems to be a novel radiological predictor of PFS [9].

2.3 Toxicity

Adverse event (AE) profile of regorafenib is similar as in the case of other tyrosine multikinase inhibitors, and the AEs of this agent are generally manageable. The most common non-hematological toxicity, which may worsen patient's quality of life, is hand-foot skin reaction (HFSR) (54%) [10–12]. Hence, many patients who experienced this AE may require treatment modification [10]. Interestingly, the incidence of HFSR seems to vary by primary tumor type. According to literature, HFSR symptoms can be found in up to 50% of regorafenib-treated patients with hepatocellular carcinoma, 60.2% of individuals with GIST, and 46.6% of persons with metastatic colorectal cancer [11]. The second most common AE in regorafenib-treated patients is arterial hypertension. Based on the data from five clinical trials, the overall incidence of arterial hypertension in regorafenib-treated patients can be estimated at 44.4% and the incidence of high-grade (G3 and higher) hypertension at 12.5%. Similar to HFSR, the risk of this AE seems to vary according to tumor type [13].

Treatment with regorafenib may also contribute to all-grade hepatotoxicity (bilirubin, AST, ALT, and ALP elevation), an AE observed in approximately one-third of patients treated with this anticancer agent [14].

Other AEs frequently associated with regorafenib treatment are oral mucositis, fatigue, nausea, weight loss, and diarrhea [12, 15]. All-grade anorexia was shown to occur more often in patients who had been previously treated with tyrosine multikinase inhibitors. On the other hand, patients from this group less commonly presented with a high-grade AST elevation [12].

The incidence of hematologic toxicities, such as thrombocytopenia, anemia, neutropenia, and leukopenia, varies between 22% (thrombocytopenia) and 13% (leukopenia). However, high-grade (G3 or higher) hematologic toxicities are relatively rarely observed in regorafenib-treated patients [16].

2.4 Regorafenib combined with other anticancer agents

In a phase I study, regorafenib combined with an anti-VEGF inhibitor, cetuximab, provided a clinical benefit, defined as the presence of stable disease or partial response. However, these promising preliminary findings need to be verified in future studies [17].

Combination therapy with regorafenib and FOLFIRI produced highly promising results, with overall disease control rate (DCR), median PFS, and median OS equal to 58.5%, 6.0 and 12.0 months, respectively [8]. An objective response rate to regorafenib combined with modified FOLFOX (mFOLFOX6) as the first-line treatment was no better than that observed in historical controls, with 85.4% DCR and median PFS of 8.5 months [18]. Negative results, specifically the lack of either OS or PFS benefit, were obtained in a study investigating the efficacy and toxicity of regorafenib plus ruxolitinib, a Janus kinase/signal transducer and activator of transcription (JAK-STAT) signaling pathway [19].

3. Trifluridine/tipiracil hydrochloride

TAS-102 is a new oral anti-metabolite drug, a 1:0.5 mixture of a thymidine-based nucleoside analog, alpha,alpha,alpha-trifluorothymidine (trifluridine: FTD), and thymidine phosphorylase inhibitor (tipiracil hydrochloride: TPI) [20–23]. FTD inhibits thymidylate synthase (TS), the key enzyme involved in DNA synthesis, whereas trifluridine incorporates into DNA via phosphorylation and initiates DNA fragmentation [20–22]. TPI enhances the exposure to FTD, improves its bioavailability, and increases the durability of response to this agent [24, 25]. Pre-exposure to 5-FU was shown to enhance FTD incorporation into DNA and to increase antitumor activity of this agent, as shown by lesser viability and proliferation of cancer cells [26]. TAS-102 proved to be effective in GI malignancies with inherent or acquired resistance to 5-FU, as well as in 5-FU-sensitive tumors [20, 21]. TAS-102 has recently been approved as the third-line treatment for adults with refractory metastatic colorectal cancer, patients with contraindications to currently available standard chemotherapy and biological therapy in the EU and USA, and individuals with unresectable advanced or recurrent colorectal cancer in Japan. The standard regimen is 35 mg/m^2 twice a day on days 1–5 and 8–12 of each 28-day cycle [24, 27].

3.1 Trials

The efficacy and safety of TAS-102 were a subject of a double-blind randomized phase II trial including Japanese patients with metastatic colorectal cancer. The patients were randomized in a 2:1 ratio to either TAS-102 or placebo arm. Median OS in the TAS-102 arm turned out to be longer than in the placebo arm (9.0 vs. 6.6 months). The most common AEs were hematologic toxicities, with grade 3 or 4 of neutropenia found in 50% of TAS-102-treated patients [28].

In a randomized double-blind phase III registration trial, TERRA, Asian patients with metastatic colorectal cancer who previously received at least two lines of systemic treatment were randomized in a 2:1 ratio to either TAS-102 or placebo group. The study confirmed the efficacy of TAS-102 in Asian population. Median OS in the TAS-102 arm was significantly longer than in the placebo group (7.8 vs. 7.1 months). Moreover, the TAS-102-treated patients had significantly lower mortality risk and significantly longer median survival follow-up time [29].

In a double-blind phase III registration trial, RECOURSE, 800 patients from Europe, North America, and Asia were randomly assigned to receive TAS-102 or placebo. PFS for the TAS-102 and placebo arm was 2.0 and 1.7 months, respectively. Patients from the TAS-102 arm had significantly longer median OS and significantly longer median time to worsening performance status (7.1 and 5.7 months, respectively) than individuals from the placebo arm (5.3 and 4.0 months, respectively). One-year OS rates for the TAS-102 and placebo arm were 27 and 18%, respectively [30]. Those promising results were further confirmed on a subgroup analysis; median OS for TAS-102-treated patients from the USA, Japan, EU, and Spain ranged between 6.5 and 7.8 months as compared with 4.3–6.7 months for the respective placebo arms, whereas median PFS in the TAS-102 and placebo groups amounted to 2.0–2.8 and 1.7–1.8 months, respectively [31, 32].

3.2 Predictors

Genetic polymorphisms in homologous recombination pathway seem to be a predictor of therapeutic response in metastatic colorectal cancer patients treated with TAS-102. According to Suenaga et al., TAS-102-treated patients with a combination of ENT1 rs760370, MATE1 rs2289669, and OCT2 rs316019 single-nucleotide polymorphisms of genes involved in trifluridine metabolism and thymidine phosphorylase inhibitor excretion had significantly longer PFS and OS [33]. Also, single-nucleotide polymorphisms of genes involved in homologous recombination, such as ATM and XRCC3, could be predictive and prognostic markers in metastatic colorectal cancer treated with TAS-102. The TAS-102-treated patients who carried any G allele in ATM rs609429 polymorphism had significantly longer OS and nonsignificantly longer PFS than carriers of the C/C variant. Also, the presence of any A allele in XRCC3 rs861539 polymorphism was shown to be associated with significantly longer OS and PFS in TAS-102-treated patients [34].

Patients with ≥ grade 2 chemotherapy-induced neutropenia (absolute neutrophil count <1500/mm^3) at 1 month (CIN-1-month) of TAS-102 therapy had longer median PFS (3.0 vs. 2.4 months) and OS (14.0 vs. 5.6 months) than those without the neutropenia. The presence of neutropenia at 1 month of TAS-102 treatment and higher baseline CEA levels were identified as independent predictors of OS [35]. In another study, grade 3 or 4 CIN-1-month was shown to be associated with longer PFS than grade 0-2 CIN-1-month (4.3 vs. 2.0 months). Moreover, G3 or G4 neutropenia during the first cycle of TAS-102 therapy turned out to be associated with significantly higher DCR (72.2%) than grade 0–2 neutropenia (72.2 vs. 30.9%) [36]. Finally, a significant association was found between baseline creatinine clearance rate of less than 57.1 mL/min prior to TAS-102 administration and the incidence of G3 or G4 neutropenia after introduction of this agent [37].

Also, longer time elapsed since the onset of the first-line therapy to disease progression (more than 18 months) seems to be a predictor of better response to TAS-102 therapy. In one study, median PFS in TAS-102-treated patients with the time to progression exceeding 18 months was longer than in those who received the first-line therapy ≤18 months before (7 vs. 5 months) [38]. These findings were later confirmed in a meta-analysis conducted by Chen et al. [39].

Kwakman et al. identified KRAS-wild type tumor, good performance status (PS0 or PS1), and normal serum levels of lactate dehydrogenase and alkaline phosphatase as independent predictors of better response to TAS-102 treatment. All these factors correlated positively with longer OS. Patients with KRAS-wild type tumors had longer median OS than those with KRAS-mutated malignancies (6.9 vs. 4.9 months), and median OS in persons with ECOG PS0–1 turned out to be longer than in individuals with worse performance status (5.9 vs. 3.2 months) [40]. However, in a meta-analysis involving the data of 1318 patients who received TAS-102, OS was significantly longer than in the study mentioned above, regardless the KRAS mutation status. Furthermore, the treatment response was not influenced by the number of metastatic sites (1, 2, or more) [39]. Also, in a subgroup analysis of patients participating in the RECOURSE trial, neither OS nor PFS correlated with the KRAS status, as well as with patients' age and ethnicity [31].

ECOG performance status (PS0 or PS1), the number of metastatic sites (1 or 2), and the time elapsed since the diagnosis of the first metastasis (18 months or longer) were identified as prognostic factors in the RECOURSE trial; however, none of those factors turned out to be a predictor of therapeutic response [30].

3.3 Toxicity

Hematologic toxicities, including leukopenia, neutropenia, and anemia, and gastrointestinal toxicities, such as nausea/vomiting, diarrhea, and the loss of appetite, as well as fatigue of various grade, were the most frequent side effects observed in patients treated with trifluridine/tipiracil [40–45]. The most common grade 3/4 toxicity was myelosuppression (neutropenia, anemia, febrile neutropenia) [46]. In turn, cardiac ischemia seems to be one of the rarest AEs observed during the therapy with TAS-102, which implies that this agent might constitute a reasonable option for patients with cardiovascular contraindications for 5-FU treatment [47].

Based on available evidence, TAS-102 seems to be a convenient, manageable, and safe agent to be used in daily clinical practice.

According to the data from the RECOURSE and J003 trials, severe AEs (SAEs) occurred in 27.7% of patients treated with TAS-102. In more than 50% of the patients, the toxicity necessitated a delay or interruption of TAS-102 therapy or dose reduction [41]. However, the incidence of SAEs and AEs leading to treatment discontinuation in TAS-102 and placebo arms was essentially similar, and fatal AEs turned out to be more common in the placebo group [41]. Furthermore, in an open-label expanded-access program, TAS-102 had similar safety profiles in older (≥65 years) and younger (<65 years) patients [48].

Finally, the occurrence of AEs had no significant impact on the quality of life and performance status of patients participating in the RECOURSE trial, even in those in whom TAS-102 had to be discontinued because of its toxicity [49].

3.4 TAS-102 combined with other anticancer drugs

In preclinical studies, TAS-102 combined with cytotoxic drugs (oxaliplatin, irinotecan) showed enhanced activity against recurrent and chemo-naïve colorectal cancers [50, 51]. Also, the regimes including TAS-102 and targeted therapies (cetuximab, panitumumab) or antiangiogenic agents (nintedanib, bevacizumab) were shown to be effective against colorectal cancer in preclinical studies [52, 53].

One phase I/II study demonstrated a promising efficacy and moderate toxicity of TAS-102 plus bevacizumab in patients with metastatic and refractory colorectal cancer [54].

The aim of currently ongoing **TR**iflUridine/tipiracil in **S**econd-line s**T**ud**Y** phase II/III study, the results of which will be available in 2022, is to determine DCR, response rate (RR), OS, PFS, safety profile, and time to treatment failure of trifluridine/tipiracil plus bevacizumab and irinotecan, fluoropyrimidine plus bevacizumab as the second-line treatments in patients with metastatic colorectal cancer who failed to respond to the first-line oxaliplatin-based therapy [55].

4. Regorafenib vs. TAS-102

An indirect comparison of regorafenib and TAS-102 based on published evidence from PubMed, Cochrane, and other databases suggests that these two agents did not differ in terms of PFS and OS benefit. However, regorafenib seems to produce all-grade toxicity more often than TAS-102 [56]. The most common forms of grade ≥3 toxicity found in regorafenib-treated patients were hepatotoxicity and palmar-plantar erythema, whereas individuals who received TAS-102 most often suffered from neutropenia [57, 58]. The similar efficacy of regorafenib and TAS-102 was confirmed in REGOTAS study (regorafenib vs. TAS-102 as salvage-line in patients with colorectal cancer refractory to standard chemotherapies: a multicenter observational study, UMIN 000020416) which showed no significant differences in OS and PFS of patients treated with one of those agents [59].

A subgroup analysis conducted within the framework of a retrospective study of Asian patients demonstrated that regorafenib was significantly more efficacious in individuals younger than 65 years, whereas TAS-102 provided greater OS benefit in persons aged 65 years or older [60]. Those findings are consistent with the results of the REGOTAS trial in which regorafenib-treated patients ≥65 years of age, with modified Glasgow Prognostic Score equal to 2 (GPS 2), had shorter OS and PFS than individuals who received TAS-102 [59]. The same study identified modified GPS before later-line chemotherapy as the strongest predictor of OS in patients with metastatic colorectal cancer [59].

Nothing has been known about the efficacy and toxicity of TAS-102 in patients treated previously with regorafenib since publication of Kotani et al.'s study. In the latter study, median PFS in patients treated with regorafenib prior to TAS-102 implementation was 2.0 months as compared with 2.1 months in individuals with no history of regorafenib treatment, and median OS in these two groups was 4.7 and 6.2 months, respectively [61]. The toxicity of TAS-102, assessed based on the incidence of at least grade 3 side effects, was similar regardless of the study group [61]. The treatment sequence analysis demonstrated that TAS-102-treated patients had longer PFS and OS after a fluoropyrimidine-based therapy-free interval, 3.1 and 17.7 months, respectively, as compared with 2.2 and 8.1 months, respectively, in persons in whom TAS-102 was implemented immediately after the fluoropyrimidine-based therapy. However, no similar association was found between the efficacy of regorafenib and the time elapsed since fluoropyrimidine-based treatment discontinuation [62].

The prognosis seems to be also influenced by the sequence of regorafenib and TAS-102 administration. Median OS in patients who received crossover treatment with regorafenib followed by TAS-102 was 11.5 months, as compared with 7.6 months in individuals in whom first TAS-102 and then regorafenib were implemented [57].

5. Re-challenge chemotherapy

Another therapeutic option in heavily pretreated patients with metastatic colorectal cancer is re-challenge chemotherapy/re-initiation chemotherapy. Re-challenge chemotherapy is defined as the re-introduction of previously used chemotherapy with oxaliplatin or irinotecan-based regimens at least 9 months after the end of the initial exposure. Re-challenge chemotherapy constitutes an important option in patients who still present with good performance status and organ function reserve, especially in those in whom the initial chemotherapy was discontinued before progression of the disease (e.g., due to cumulative toxicities) [63–65]. Such approach did not shorten the period of the best supportive care and, more importantly, might prolong OS [65]. According to Chambers et al., clinical benefit rate (defined as the proportion of patients with partial response or stable disease) after re-challenge chemotherapy was 75.5% and time to progression equaled 6.5 months [63]. Moreover, re-challenge chemotherapy after regorafenib treatment seems to be a good strategy in heavily pretreated patients with metastatic colorectal cancer. According to literature, PFS after re-challenge chemotherapy varied between 0.5 and 3.5 months, and 6-month OS reached up to 27.3%. In some researchers' opinion, regorafenib could resensitize cancer patients to previously given chemotherapy, but this hypothesis still needs to be verified empirically [66].

Some authors reported the use of re-initiation chemotherapy or second re-challenge chemotherapy after the development of resistance, but none of these approaches is a standard of oncological treatment [63, 64].

6. Combination of capecitabine and mitomycin C (MMC)

MMC is a cytotoxic antibiotic which shows moderate efficacy when used as monotherapy in colorectal cancer patients. Upregulation of intra-tumoral thymidine phosphorylase, an enzyme converting capecitabine to 5-FU, is the primary mechanism through which MMC acts synergistically to capecitabine [67]. According to literature, overall response rate in patients with metastatic colorectal cancer who received MMC (6 mg/m^2 intravenously on day 1 every 3 weeks) plus capecitabine (1000 mg/m^2 twice daily on days 1–14, followed by a 7-day treatment-free interval) ranged between 15.2 and 55.5% [68–72]. The majority of patients received previously two, three, or even four lines of anticancer therapy. Median PFS varied between 1.7 and 5.4 months [68–71, 74] and median OS between 5.4 and 13 months [68–72, 74]. While those results might be considered disappointing, it should be emphasized that all patients were pretreated with many lines of systemic therapy and had metastases in multiple locations.

With no doubt, the combination therapy with capecitabine and MMC is dedicated primarily for patients with cumulative side effects after previous treatment and/or contraindications to targeted therapies [70]. Furthermore, capecitabine plus MMC constitutes a good option of the best supportive care in patients who still maintain good performance status and organ efficiency, especially in countries in which regorafenib and TAS-102 have been registered but are not reimbursed.

Toxicity of capecitabine plus MMC combination is mild, acceptable, and easily manageable, and no significant hematological AEs have been reported thus far [71, 73–74]. The main non-hematological AEs documented in patients treated with this regimen are palmar-plantar erythema, nausea, diarrhea, and fatigue [71, 73–74].

7. Conclusions

Regorafenib and trifluridine/tipiracil have been authorized for the treatment of metastatic colorectal cancer, as the third or further therapy line. The patients are eligible for one of those treatments if they present with good performance status and adequate bone marrow, liver, and kidney function; hence, aside from clinical and molecular biomarker status, also those factors should be considered during patient qualification. While the toxicity of both anticancer agents is manageable, appropriate control of side effects requires clinical vigilance and good medication compliance. In some clinical situations, re-induction/re-challenge of previously given chemotherapy with oxaliplatin or irinotecan-based regimens and/or switching to mitomycin C plus capecitabine might be a reasonable option.

Conflict of interest

The author declares no conflict of interest.

Author details

Aneta L. Zygulska
Department of Oncology, University Hospital in Krakow, Poland

*Address all correspondence to: zygulska@poczta.onet.pl

References

[1] Strumberg D, Schultheis B. Regorafenib for cancer. Expert Opinion on Investigational Drugs. 2012;**21**:879-889. DOI: 10.1517/13543784.2012.684752

[2] Crona DJ, Keisler MD, Walko CM. Regorafenib: A novel multitargeted tyrosine kinase inhibitor for colorectal cancer and gastrointestinal stromal tumors. The Annals of Pharmacotherapy. 2013;**47**:1685-1696. DOI: 10.1177/1060028013509792

[3] Grothey A, Van Cutsem E, Sobrero A, Siena S, Falcone A, Ychou M, et al. Regorafenib monotherapy for previously treated metastatic colorectal cancer (CORRECT): An international, multicentre, randomised, placebo-controlled, phase 3 trial. Lancet. 2013;**381**(9863):303-312. DOI: 10.1016/S0140-6736(12)61900-X

[4] Li J, Qin S, Xu R, Yau TC, Ma B, Pan H, et al. Regorafenib plus best supportive care versus placebo plus best supportive care in Asian patients with previously treated metastatic colorectal cancer (CONCUR): A randomised, double-blind, placebo-controlled, phase 3 trial. The Lancet Oncology. 2015;**16**:619-629. DOI: 10.1016/S1470-2045(15)70156-7

[5] Garcia-Alonso P, Benavides M, Falco E, Munoz A, Gomez A, Sastre J, et al. Single-agent regorafenib in metastatic colorectal cancer patients with any RAS or BRAF mutation previously treated with FOLFOXIRI plus bevacizumab (PREVIUM trial). The Oncologist. 2018;**23**:1271-e128. DOI: 10.1634/theoncologist.2018-0316

[6] Komori A, Taniguchi H, Hamauchi S, Masuishi T, Kito Y, Narita Y, et al. Serum CA19-9 response is an early predictive marker of efficacy of regorafenib in refractory metastatic colorectal cancer. Oncology. 2017;**93**:329-335. DOI: 10.1159/000479280

[7] Tabernero J, Lenz HJ, Siena S, Soobrero A, Falcone A, Ychou M, et al. Analysis of circulating DNA and protein biomarkers to predict the clinical activity of regorafenib and assess prognosis in patients with metastatic colorectal cancer: A retrospective, exploratory analysis of the CORRECT trial. The Lancet Oncology. 2015;**16**:937-948. DOI: 10.1016/S1470-2045(15)00138-2

[8] Ma CJ, Huang CW, Chang TK, Tsai HL, Su WC, Yeh YS, et al. Oncologic outcomes in metastatic colorectal cancer with regorafenib with FOLFIRI as a third- or fourth-line setting. Translational Oncology. 2018;**12**(3):502-512. DOI: 10.1016/j.tranon.2018.12.003

[9] Ricotta R, Verrioli A, Ghezzi S, Porcu L, Grothey A, Falcone A, et al. Radiological imaging markers predicting clinical outcome in patients with metastatic colorectal carcinoma treated with regorafenib: Post hoc analysis of the CORRECT phase III trial (RadioCORRECT study). ESMO Open. 2017;**1**(6):e000111. DOI: 10.1136/esmoopen-2016-000111

[10] McLellan B, Ciardiello F, Lacouture ME, Segaert S, Van Cutsem E. Regorafenib-associated hand-foot skin reaction: Practical advice on diagnosis, prevention, and management. Annals of Oncology. 2015;**26**:2017-2026. DOI: 10.1093/annonc/mdv244

[11] Belum VR, Wu S, Lacouture ME. Risk of hand-foot skin reaction with the novel multikinase inhibitor regorafenib: A meta-analysis. Investigational New Drugs. 2013;**31**:1078-1086. DOI: 10.1007/s10637-013-9977-0

[12] Yin X, Yin Y, Shen C, Chen H, Wang J, Cai Z, et al. Adverse events risk associated with regorafenib in the treatment of advanced solid tumors:

Meta-analysis of randomized controlled trials. OncoTargets and Therapy. 2018;**11**:6405-6414. DOI: 10.2147/OTT.S156760

[13] Wang Z, Xu J, Nie W, Huang G, Tang J, Guan X. Risk of hypertension with regorafenib in cancer patients: A systematic review and meta-analysis. European Journal of Clinical Pharmacology. 2014;**70**:225-231. DOI: 10.1007/s00228-013-1598-1

[14] Zhao B, Zhao H. Incidence and risk of regorafenib-induced hepatotoxicity. Oncotarget. 2017;**8**:84102-84111. DOI: 10.18632/oncotarget.21106

[15] Grothey A, George S, van Cutsem E, Blay JY, Sobrero A, Demetri GD. Optimizing treatment outcomes with regorafenib: Personalized dosing and other strategies to support patient care. The Oncologist. 2014;**19**:669-680. DOI: 10.1634/theoncologist.2013-0059

[16] Zhao B, Zhao H. Incidence and risk of hematologic toxicities in cancer patients treated with regorafenib. Oncotarget. 2017;**8**:93813-93824. DOI: 10.18632/oncotarget.21217

[17] Subbiah V, Khawaja MR, Homg DS, Amini B, Yungfang J, Liu H, et al. First-in-human trial of multikinase VEGF inhibitor regorafenib and anti-EGFR antibody cetuximab in advanced cancer patients. JCI Insight. 2017;**2**:90380. DOI: 10.1172/jci.insight.90380

[18] Argiles G, Saunders MP, Rivera F, Sobrero A, Benson A 3rd, Guillen Ponce C, et al. Regorafenib plus modified FOLFOX6 as first-line treatment of metastatic colorectal cancer: A phase II trial. European Journal of Cancer. 2015;**51**:942-949. DOI: 10.1016/j.ejca.2015.02.013

[19] Fogelman D, Cubillo A, Garcia-Alfonso P, Miron MLL, Nemunaitis J, Flora D, et al. Randomized, double-blind, phase two study of ruxolitinib plus regorafenib in patients with relapsed/refractory metastatic colorectal cancer. Cancer Medicine. 2018;7:5382-5393. DOI: 10.1002/cam4.1703

[20] Emura T, Murakami Y, Nakagawa F, Fukushima M, Kitazato K. A novel antimetabolite, TAS-102 retains its effect on FU-related resistant cancer cells. International Journal of Molecular Medicine. 2004;**13**:545-549

[21] Emura T, Suzuki N, Yamaguchi M, Ohshimo H, Fukushima M. A novel combination antimetabolite, TAS-102, exhibits antitumor activity in FU-resistant human cancer cells through a mechanism involving FTD incorporation in DNA. International Journal of Oncology. 2004;**25**:571-578

[22] Miyamoto Y, Lenz HJ, Baba H. A novel antimetabolite: TAS-102 for metastatic colorectal cancer. Expert Review of Clinical Pharmacology. 2016;**9**:355-365. DOI: 10.1586/17512433.2016.1133285

[23] Zaniboni A, Bertocchi P, Barni S, Petrelli F. TAS-102 (Lonsurf) for the treatment of metastatic colorectal cancer. A concise review. Clinical Colorectal Cancer. 2016;**15**:292-297. DOI: 10.1016/j.clcc.2016.06.003

[24] Burness CB, Duggan ST. Trifluridine/tipiracil: A review in metastatic colorectal cancer. Drugs. 2016;**76**:1393-1402. DOI: 10.1007/s40265-016-0633-9

[25] Lenz HJ, Stintzing S, Loupakis F. TAS-102, a novel antitumor agent: A review of the mechanism of action. Cancer Treatment Reviews. 2015;**41**:777-783. DOI: 10.1016/j.ctrv.2015.06.001

[26] Baba T, Kokuryo T, Yamaguchi J, Yokoyama Y, Uehara K, Ebata T, et al. Pre-exposure to fluorouracil increased trifluridine incorporation and enhanced its anti-tumor effect for

colorectal cancer. Anticancer Research. 2018;**38**:1427-1434

[27] Peeters M, Cervantes A, Moreno Vera S, Taieb J. Trifluridine/tipiracil: An emerging strategy for the management of gastrointestinal cancers. Future Oncology. 2018;**14**:1629-1645. DOI: 10.2217/fon-2018-0147

[28] Yoshino T, Mizunuma N, Yamazaki K, Nishina T, Komatsu Y, Baba H, et al. TAS-102 monotherapy for pretreated metastatic colorectal cancer: A double-blind, randomised, placebo-controlled phase 2 trial. The Lancet Oncology. 2012;**13**:993-1001. DOI: 10.1016/S1470-2045(12)70345-5

[29] Xu J, Kim TW, Shen L, Sriuranpong V, Pan H, Xu R, et al. Results of a randomized, double-blind, placebo-controlled, phase III trial of trifluridine/tipiracil (TAS-102) monotherapy in Asian patients with previously treated metastatic colorectal cancer: The TERRA study. Journal of Clinical Oncology. 2018;**36**:350-358. DOI: 10.1200/JCO.2017.74.3245

[30] Mayer RJ, Van Cutsem E, Falcone A, Yoshino T, Garcia-Carbonero R, Mizunuma N, et al. Randomized trial of TAS-102 for refractory metastatic colorectal cancer. The New England Journal of Medicine. 2015;**372**:1909-1919. DOI: 10.1056/NEJMoa1414325

[31] Van Cutsem E, Mayer RJ, Laurent S, Winkler R, Gravalos C, Benavides M, et al. The subgroups of the phase III RECOURSE trial of trifluridine/tipiracil (TAS-102) versus placebo with best supportive care in patients with metastatic colorectal cancer. European Journal of Cancer. 2018;**90**:63-72. DOI: 10.1016/j.ejca.2017.10.009

[32] Longo-Munoz F, Argiles G, Tabernero J, Cervantes A, Gravalos C, Pericay C, et al. Efficacy of trifluridine and tipiracil (TAS-102) versus placebo, with supportive care, in a randomized, controlled trial of patients with metastatic colorectal cancer from Spain: Results of a subgroup analysis of the phase 3 RECOURSE trial. Clinical & Translational Oncology. 2017;**19**:227-235. DOI: 10.1007/s12094-016-1528-7

[33] Suenaga M, Schirripa M, Cao S, Zhang W, Yang D, Dadduzio V, et al. Potential role of polymorphisms in the transporter genes ENT1 and MATE1/OCT2 in predicting TAS-102 efficacy and toxicity in patients with refractory metastatic colorectal cancer. European Journal of Cancer. 2017;**86**:197-206. DOI: 10.1016/j.ejca.2017.08.033

[34] Suenaga M, Schirripa M, Cao S, Zhang W, Yang D, Murgioni S, et al. Genetic variants of DNA repair-related genes predict efficacy of TAS-102 in patients with refractory metastatic colorectal cancer. Annals of Oncology. 2017;**28**:1015-1022. DOI: 10.1093/annonc/mdx035

[35] Kasi PM, Kotani D, Cecchini M, Shitara K, Ohtsu A, Ramanathan RK, et al. Chemotherapy induced neutropenia at 1-month mark is a predictor of overall survival in patients receiving TAS-102 for refractory metastatic colorectal cancer: A cohort study. BMC Cancer. 2016;**16**:467. DOI: 10.1186/s12885-016-2491-y

[36] Hamauchi S, Yamazaki K, Masuishi T, Kito Y, Komori A, Tsushima T, et al. Neutropenia as a predictive factor in metastatic colorectal cancer treated with TAS-102. Clinical Colorectal Cancer. 2017;**16**:51-57. DOI: 10.1016/j.clcc.2016.07.005

[37] Yasue F, Kimura M, Usami E, Iwai M, Kawachi S, Mitsuoka M, et al. Risk factors contributing to the development of neutropenia in patients receiving oral trifluridine-tipiracil (TAS-102) chemotherapy for advanced/recurrent colorectal cancer. Die Pharmazie. 2018;**73**:178-181. DOI: 10.1691/ph.2018.7908

[38] Skuja E, Gerina-Berzina A, Hegmane A, Zvirbule Z, Vecvagare E, Purkalne G. Duration of previous treatment as a prognostic factor in metastatic colorectal cancer treated with trifluridine/tipiracil. Molecular and Clinical Oncology. 2018;**8**:699-702. DOI: 10.3892/mco.2018.1600

[39] Chen D, Wu YS, lin H, Wang Y, Li L, Zhang T. Efficacy and safety of TAS-102 in refractory metastatic colorectal cancer: A meta-analysis. Cancer Management and Research. 2018;**10**:2915-2924. DOI: 10.2147/CMAR.S174584

[40] Kwakman JJM, Vink G, Vestjens JH, Beerepoot LV, de Groot JW, Jansen RL, et al. Feasibility and effectiveness of trifluridine/tipiracil in metastatic colorectal cancer: Real-life data from the Netherlands. International Journal of Clinical Oncology. 2018;**23**:482-489. DOI: 10.1007/s10147-017-1220-0

[41] Falcone A, Ohtsu A, Van Cutsem E, Mayer RJ, Buscaglia M, Bendell JC, et al. Integrated safety summary for trifluridine/tipiracil (TAS-102). Anti-Cancer Drugs. 2018;**29**:89-96. DOI: 10.1097/CAD.0000000000000554

[42] Lee JJ, Chu E. Adherence, dosing, and managing toxicities with trifluridine/tipiracil (TAS-102). Clinical Colorectal Cancer. 2017;**16**:85-92. DOI: 10.1016/j.clcc.2017.01.003

[43] White T, Larson H, Minnella A, Hochster HS. Metastatic colorectal cancer: Management with trifluridine/tipiracil. Clinical Journal of Oncology Nursing. 2017;**21**:E30-E37. DOI: 10.1188/17.CJON.E30-E37

[44] Kasper S, Kisro J, Fuchs M, Muller C, Schulz-Abelius A, Karthaus M, et al. Safety profile of trifluridine/tipiracil monotherapy in clinical practice: Results of the German compassionate-use program for patients with metastatic colorectal cancer. BMC Cancer. 2018;**18**:1124. DOI: 10.1186/s12885-018-5063-5

[45] Overman MJ, Kopetz S, Varadhachary G, Fukushima M, Kuwata K, Mita A, et al. Phase I clinical study of three times a day oral administration of TAS-102 in patients with solid tumors. Cancer Investigation. 2008;**26**:794-799. DOI: 10.1080/07357900802087242

[46] Bendell JC, Rosen LS, Mayer RJ, Goldman JW, Infante JR, Benedetti F, et al. Phase 1 study of oral TAS-102 in patients with refractory metastatic colorectal cancer. Cancer Chemotherapy and Pharmacology. 2015;**76**:925-932. DOI: 10.1007/s00280-015-2850-4

[47] Vaflard P, Ederhy S, Torregrosa C, Andre T, Cohen R, Lopez-Trabada D. Fluoropyrimidines cardiac toxicity: 5-Fluorouracil, capecitabine, compound S-1 and trifluridine/tipiracil. Bulletin du Cancer. 2018;**105**:707-719. DOI: 10.1016/j.bulcan.2018.05.005

[48] Mayer RJ, Hochster HS, Cohen SJ, Winkler R, Makris L, Grothey A. Safety of trifluridine/tipiracil in an open-label expanded-access program in elderly and younger patients with metastatic colorectal cancer. Cancer Chemotherapy and Pharmacology. 2018;**82**:961-969. DOI: 10.1007/s00280-018-3686-5

[49] Van Cutsem E, Falcone A, Garcia-Carbonero R, Komatsu Y, Pastorino A, Peeters M, et al. Proxies of quality of life in metastatic colorectal cancer: Analyses in the RECOURSE trial. ESMO Open. 2017;**2**:e000261. DOI: 10.1136/esmoopen-2017-000261

[50] Nukatsuka M, Nakagawa F, Takechi T. Efficacy of combination chemotherapy using a novel oral chemotherapeutic agent, TAS-102, with oxaliplatin on human colorectal and gastric cancer xenografts. Anticancer Research. 2015;**35**:4605-4615

[51] Nukatsuka M, Nakagawa F, Saito H, Sakata M, Uchida J, Takechi T. Efficacy of combination chemotherapy using a novel oral chemotherapeutic agent, TAS-102, with irinotecan hydrochloride on human colorectal and gastric cancer xenografts. Anticancer Research. 2015;**35**:1437-1445

[52] Tsukihara H, Nakagawa F, Sakamoto K, Ishida K, Tanaka N, Okabe H, et al. Efficacy of combination chemotherapy using a novel oral chemotherapeutic agent, TAS-102, together with bevacizumab, cetuximab, or panitumumab on human colorectal cancer xenografts. Oncology Reports. 2015;**33**:2135-2142. DOI: 10.3892/or.2015.3876

[53] Suzuki N, Nakagawa F, Matsuoka K, Takechi T. Effect of a novel oral chemotherapeutic agent containing a combination of trifluridine, tipiracil and the novel triple angiokinase inhibitor nintedanib, on human colorectal cancer xenografts. Oncology Reports. 2016;**36**:3123-3130. DOI: 10.3892/or.2016.5208

[54] Kuboki Y, Nishina T, Shinozaki E, Yamazaki K, Shitara K, Okamoto W, et al. TAS-102 plus bevacizumab for patients with metastatic colorectal cancer refractory to standard therapies (C-TASK FORCE): An investigator-initiated, open-label, single-arm, multicentre, phase 1/2 study. The Lancet Oncology. 2017;**18**:1172-1181. DOI: 10.1016/S1470-2045(17)30425-4

[55] Yoshino T, Oki E, Nozawa H, Eguchi-Nakajima T, Taniguchi H, Morita S, et al. Open rationale and design of the TRUSTY study: A randomised, multicentre, open-label phase II/III study of trifluridine/tipiracil plus bevacizumab versus irinotecan, fluoropyrimidine plus bevacizumab as second-line treatment in patients with metastatic colorectal cancer progressive during or following first-line oxaliplatin-based chemotherapy. ESMO Open. 2018;**3**:e000411. DOI: 10.1136/esmoopen-2018-000411

[56] Abrahao ABK, Ko YJ, Berry S, Chan KKW. A comparison of regorafenib and TAS-102 for metastatic colorectal cancer: A systematic review and network meta-analysis. Clinical Colorectal Cancer. 2018;**17**:113-120. DOI: 10.1016/j.clcc.2017.10.016

[57] Sueda T, Sakai D, Kudo T, Sugiura T, Takahashi H, Haraguchi N, et al. Efficacy and safety of regorafenib or TAS-102 in patients with metastatic colorectal cancer refractory to standard therapies. Anticancer Research. 2016;**36**:4299-4306

[58] Masuishi T, Taniguchi H, Hamauchi S, Komori A, Kito Y, Narita Y, et al. Regorafenib versus trifluridine/tipiracil for refractory metastatic colorectal cancer: A retrospective comparison. Clinical Colorectal Cancer. 2017;**16**:e15-e22. DOI: 10.1016/j.clcc.2016.07.019

[59] Tsuchihashi K, Ito M, Moriwaki T, Fukuoka S, Taniguchi H, Takashima A, et al. Role of predictive value of the modified Glasgow prognostic score for later-line chemotherapy in patients with metastatic colorectal cancer. Clinical Colorectal Cancer. 2018;**17**:e687-e697. DOI: 10.1016/j.clcc.2018.07.004

[60] Moriwaki T, Fukuoka S, Taniguchi H, Takashima A, Kumekawa Y, Kajiwara T, et al. Propensity score analysis of regorafenib versus trifluridine/tipiracil in patients with metastatic colorectal cancer refractory to standard chemotherapy (REGOTAS): A Japanese society for cancer of the colon and rectum multicenter observational study. The Oncologist. 2018;**23**:7-15. DOI: 10.1634/theoncologist.2017-0275

[61] Kotani D, Shitara K, Kawazoe A, Fukuoka S, Kuboki Y, Bando H, et al. Safety and efficacy of trifluridine/tipiracil monotherapy in clinical practice for patients with metastatic

colorectal cancer: Experience at a single institution. Clinical Colorectal Cancer. 2016;**15**:e109-e115. DOI: 10.1016/j.clcc.2015.11.005

[62] Unseld M, Drimmel M, Siebenhuner A, Gleiss A, Bianconi D, Kieler M, et al. Optimizing treatment sequence for late-line metastatic colorectal cancer patients using trifluridine/tipiracil and regorafenib. Clinical Colorectal Cancer. 2018;**17**:274-279. DOI: 10.1016/j.clcc.2018.05.012

[63] Chambers AE, Frick J, Tanner N, Gerkin R, Kundranda M, Dragovich T. Chemotherapy re-challenge response rate in metastatic colorectal cancer. Journal of Gastrointestinal Oncology. 2018;**9**:679-686. DOI: 10.21037/jgo.2018.04.08

[64] Vogel A, Hofheinz RD, Kubicka S, Arnold D. Treatment decisions in metastatic colorectal cancer—Beyond first and second line combination therapies. Cancer Treatment Reviews. 2017;**59**:54-60. DOI: 10.1016/j.ctrv.2017.04.007

[65] Takeuchi N, Koike K, Yoshida S, Kudo A, Sekiguchi N, Nakayama A, et al. Treatment of metastatic refractory colorectal cancer following regorafenib failure. Molecular and Clinical Oncology. 2017;**7**:308-312. DOI: 10.3892/mco.2017.1307

[66] Bertocchi P, Aroldi F, Prochilo T, Meriggi F, Beretta GD, Zaniboni A. Chemotherapy rechallenge after regorafenib treatment in metastatic colorectal cancer: Still hope after the last hope? Journal of Chemotherapy. 2017;**29**:102-105. DOI: 10.1080/1120009X.2016.1247205

[67] Sawada N, Ishikawa T, Fukase Y, Nishida M, Yoshikubo T, Ishitsuka H. Induction of thymidine phosphorylase activity and enhancement of capcitabine efficacy by taxol/taxotere in human cancer xenografts. Clinical Cancer Research. 1998;**4**:1013-1019

[68] Vdorljak E, Omrcen T, Boban M, Hrepic D. Capecitabine and mitomycin-C in the therapy of pretreated patients with metastatic colorectal cancer: Single center retrospective study with 36 patients. Journal of BUON. 2008;**13**:513-518

[69] Chong G, Dickson JLB, Cunningham D, Norman AR, Rao S, Hill ME, et al. Capecitabine and mitomycin C as third-line therapy for patients with metastatic colorectal cancer resistant to fluorouracil and irinotecan. British Journal of Cancer. 2005;**93**:510-514

[70] Rimassal L, Gullo G, Carnaghi C, Abbadessa G, Zuradelli M, Tronconi MC, et al. Chemotherapy with mitomycin C and capecitabine in patients with advanced colorectal cancer pretreated with irinotecan and oxaliplatin. Tumori. 2006;**92**:285-289

[71] Scartozzi M, Falcone A, Fucci F, Braconi C, Pierantoni C, Cavanna L, et al. Capecitabine and mitomycin C may be an effective treatment option for third-line chemotherapy in advanced colorectal cancer. Tumori. 2006;**92**:384-388

[72] Saif MW, Kaley K, Brennan M, Garcon MC, Rodriguez G. Mitomycin-C and capecitabine (MIXE) as salvage treatment in patients with refractory, metastatic colorectal cancer: A retrospective study. Anticancer Research. 2013;**33**:2743-2746

[73] Ferrarotto R, Machado K, Mak MP, Shah N, Takahashi TK, Costa FP, et al. Multicenter, multinational analysis of mitomycin C in refractory metastatic colorectal cancer. European Journal of Cancer. 2012;**48**:820-826

[74] Zygulska AL, Krzemieniecki K. Salvage chemotherapy in metastatic colorectal cancer with the combination of capeitabine and mitomycin C. Neoplasma. 2015;**62**:793-797